Diagnosis and Treatment of Mycobacterial Infections

Edited by Liang Wang, Lijun Bi, Xuejiao Hu and Yudong Zhang

Published in London, United Kingdom

Diagnosis and Treatment of Mycobacterial Infections
http://dx.doi.org/10.5772/intechopen.1005549
Edited by Liang Wang, Lijun Bi, Xuejiao Hu and Yudong Zhang

Contributors
Axhell Aleid Cornejo-Báez, Chao Gao, Fen Li, Gowsalya Saminathan, Jian-Song Gu, Jin-Bin Fan, Julieta Luna-Herrera, Jumei Zeng, Karen Delgadillo-Gutiérrez, Karolina D. Witt, Liang Wang, Qin-Hui Zhu, Radha Gopalaswamy, Sinazo Cobongela, Siva Kumar Shanmugam, Ting-Ting Huang, Tintswalo Mgwenya, Vasudevan Manoharan, Xiao Zhao, Xingyan Tan, Xue-Song Xiong, Yi-Wen Liao, Yu-Rong Qin, Zhan-Zhong Liu

First published in London, United Kingdom, 2025 by IntechOpen
IntechOpen is the global imprint of INTECHOPEN LIMITED, registered in England and Wales, registration number: 11086078, 167-169 Great Portland Street, London, W1W 5PF, United Kingdom

For EU product safety concerns: IN TECH d.o.o., Prolaz Marije Krucifikse Kozulić 3, 51000 Rijeka, Croatia, info@intechopen.com or visit our website at intechopen.com.

British Library Cataloguing-in-Publication Data
A catalogue record for this book is available from the British Library

Diagnosis and Treatment of Mycobacterial Infections
Edited by Liang Wang, Lijun Bi, Xuejiao Hu and Yudong Zhang
p. cm.
Print ISBN 978-1-83634-278-6
Online ISBN 978-1-83634-277-9
eBook (PDF) ISBN 978-1-83634-279-3

Meet the editors

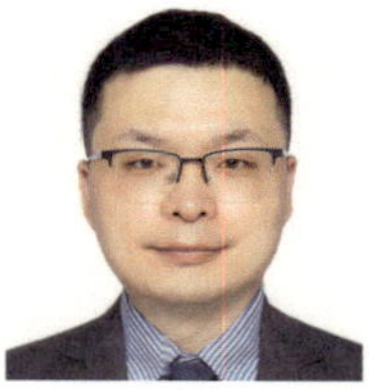

Liang Wang is a Full Professor and a Senior Medical Research Fellow. He serves as an Associate Editor for Frontiers in Microbiology and Gene Reports, and an editorial board member for BMC Microbiology and PeerJ. Prof. Wang has published over 150 peer-reviewed papers in international journals, including Lancet Microbe, npj Digital Medicine, Trends in Analytical Chemistry, and ISME Journal. He received the 2025 Rising Star Award in Measurement Science from the American Chemical Society and is frequently invited to give presentations and chair sessions at domestic and international conferences such as ICPNFF (Hong Kong, China, 2025), CHRO (Perth, Australia, 2024), and VAAM (Gottingen, Germany, 2023), etc.

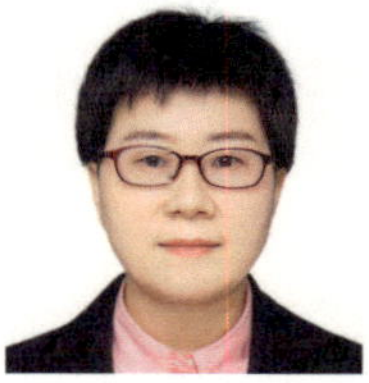

Lijun Bi, Ph.D., is a Professor and Ph.D. Supervisor at Guangzhou National Laboratory (GZNL) since 2022. She is also a Supervisor at the Institute of Biophysics, Chinese Academy of Sciences. Dr. Bi has served as the Deputy Director of the CAS Key Laboratory of Non-coding RNA and Director of the Foshan Branch of the CAS Institute of Biophysics (2013-2021), as well as former Associate Director of the CAS Institute of Biophysics. Her primary focus is on research and innovation in TB systems biology and translational medicine.

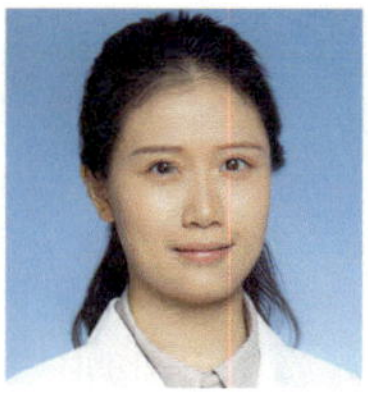

Xuejiao Hu, Ph.D., has been an Associate Chief Technician at the Laboratory of Medicine, Guangdong Provincial People's Hospital (Guangdong Academy of Medical Sciences), Southern Medical University since 2020. She has dedicated her work to translational research on the interaction between MTB and its host, as well as biomarker screening for TB diseases.

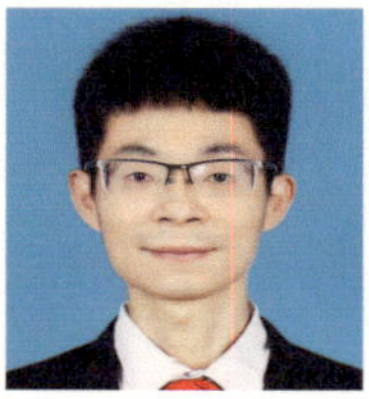

Dr. Yu-Dong Zhang is a lecturer at the First School of Clinical Medicine at Xuzhou Medical University. He graduated from the School of Public Health, Xuzhou Medical University, majoring in preventive medicine. He received his master's degree from the School of Public Health of Nanjing Medical University. During this period, he conducted toxicology research at the Key Laboratory of Toxicology, a Ministry of Education institution. He has published more than 10 academic papers, one of which was among the Top 10 excellent papers of the year, as selected by the American Society of Toxicology. He serves as a reviewer for journals such as the International Journal of Neuroscience. He has led three scientific research projects focusing on clinical epidemiology.

Contents

Preface

Mycobacteria are a group of bacteria including pathogenic and non-pathogenic species, among which pathogenic mycobacterial species can cause a series of diseases in human beings, mainly including tuberculosis (TB) caused by *Mycobacterium tuberculosis* (Mtb), leprosy caused by *Mycobacterium leprae*, and infections caused by nontuberculous mycobacteria (NTM) [1]. According to the List of Prokaryotic Names with Standing in Nomenclature (LPSN), the genus *Mycobacterium* comprises 195 recognized and validly published species. However, new species are continuously being identified, especially for nontuberculous species [2]. According to the latest data from the World Health Organization, approximately one-quarter of the global population has been infected with TB bacteria. In 2023 alone, around 10.8 million people fell ill with TB all over the world, with 1.25 million people succumbing to tuberculosis, which made the infection the world's leading cause of death due to a single infectious agent. As for NTM, they are a group of opportunistic bacterial pathogens that commonly infect hosts, particularly in the elderly and immunocompromised population, via inhalation and skin contact with the environment [1]. A recent retrospective observational study reported that the number of NTM infection-related deaths in 83 countries was 42,182 between 2000 and 2022, based on the data from the mortality database of the WHO, and 86% of deaths occurred in people aged 65 years or older [3]. Considering the increasing prevalence of mycobacterial infections, early diagnosis and targeted treatment are crucial for managing and reducing the corresponding mortality.

Multiple methods have been developed for diagnosing mycobacterial infections, including smear microscopy, bacterial culture, serological tests, immunological assays, molecular techniques, and chest X-ray screening [4, 5]. However, these regular methods suffer from certain limitations, including testing inaccuracy and a long turnaround time. Recent advancements in technology have led to the development of innovative methods for detecting bacterial infections, including digital droplet PCR [6], whole-genome sequencing [7], and Raman spectroscopy [8, 9]. These techniques demonstrate significant potential for the rapid and precise diagnosis of mycobacterial infections, owing to their low sample volume requirements, high-throughput capabilities, and enhanced detection sensitivity. It is worth noting that NTM prevalence has been rising [10]. However, due to the similar symptoms of Mtb and NTM, such as cough, fever, and weight loss, it is challenging to distinguish between the two types of mycobacterial infections, particularly in resource-limited settings with insufficient testing capacities, leading to misdiagnosis and mistreatment [10]. Therefore, innovative techniques and advanced technologies are urgently needed to deliver faster, more cost-effective, and highly accurate outcomes in combating highly transmissible infections.

As such, we have edited this book, *Diagnosis and Treatment of Mycobacterial Infections*. This edited book contains chapters written by international teams, including basic and clinical experts from China, Mexico, the United Kingdom, South Africa, and other countries. These chapters provide advanced knowledge and updated information on mycobacterial pathogenesis, drug resistance, diagnosis, and treatment strategies for relevant students, researchers, healthcare professionals, and other interested readers, facilitating an understanding of mycobacterial species and enabling the accurate diagnosis and effective treatment of mycobacterial infections. With the development of novel diagnostic methods and treatment strategies, the infection rate and mortality of mycobacterial infections are expected to be significantly reduced in the future.

Editing this book has been a journey, and we extend our deepest gratitude to those who accompanied us along the way. We extend our heartfelt thanks to the exceptional team at IntechOpen, particularly Publishing Process Manager Mr. Josip Knapic and Commissioning Editor Filip Lovricevic, for their insightful feedback, unwavering patience, and steadfast support throughout the process. We are equally grateful to the talented authors of the book chapters, whose expertise and dedication brought this project to life, and to our readers, whose curiosity and engagement inspire us to continue this work.

Liang Wang
Department of Intelligent Medical Engineering,
School of Medical Informatics and Engineering,
Xuzhou Medical University,
Xuzhou, Jiangsu Province, China

Guangdong Provincial People's Hospital,
Guangdong Academy of Medical Sciences,
Southern Medical University,
Guangzhou, Guangdong Province, China

Lijun Bi
Guangzhou National Laboratory,
Guangzhou, Guangdong Province, China

Xuejiao Hu
Guangdong Provincial People's Hospital,
Guangdong Academy of Medical Sciences,
Southern Medical University,
Guangzhou, Guangdong Province, China

Yudong Zhang
The First School of Clinical Medicine,
Xuzhou Medical University,
Xuzhou, Jiangsu Province, China

References

[1] Tutumlu TK, Dollé C, Kusejko K, et al. Mycobacteria beyond disease. *Trends in Microbiology.* 2025.

[2] Armstrong DT, Eisemann E, Parrish N, Humphries RM. A Brief Update on Mycobacterial Taxonomy, 2020 to 2022. *Journal of Clinical Microbiology.* 2023;61(4).

[3] Harada K, Vu QT, Nishimura Y, et al. Trends in nontuberculous mycobacterial disease mortality based on 2000-2022 data from 83 countries. *International Journal of Infectious Diseases.* 2025;158.

[4] Ying C, Zhang L, Jin X, Zhu D, Wu W. Advances in diagnosis and treatment of non-tuberculous mycobacterial lung disease. *Diagnostic Microbiology and Infectious Disease.* 2024;109(2).

[5] Wang L, Zhang X-D, Tang J-W, et al. Machine learning analysis of SERS fingerprinting for the rapid determination of Mycobacterium tuberculosis infection and drug resistance. *Computational and Structural Biotechnology Journal.* 2022;20:5364-5377.

[6] Kitagawa H, Kojima M, Tadera K, et al. Clinical diagnostic performance of droplet digital PCR for pathogen detection in patients with Escherichia coli bloodstream infection: a prospective observational study. *BMC Infectious Diseases.* 2025;25(1).

[7] Wilkinson H, McDonald J, McCarthy HS, et al. Using nanopore sequencing to identify bacterial infection in joint replacements: a preliminary study. *Briefings in Functional Genomics.* 2024;23(5):509-516.

[8] Tang J-W, Yuan Q, Zhang L, Marshall BJ, Yen Tay AC, Wang L. Application of machine learning-assisted surface-enhanced Raman spectroscopy in medical laboratories: Principles, opportunities, and challenges. *TrAC Trends in Analytical Chemistry.* 2025;184.

[9] Tang JW, Yuan Q, Wen XR, Usman M, Tay ACY, Wang L. Label-free surface-enhanced Raman spectroscopy coupled with machine learning algorithms in pathogenic microbial identification: Current trends, challenges, and perspectives. *Interdisciplinary Medicine.* 2024;2(3).

[10] Anand AR, Biswas J. TB or NTM: Can a new multiplex PCR assay be the answer? *eBioMedicine.* 2021;71.

Section 1

Overview of Mycobacterial Infections

Chapter 1

Comparative Genomics of *Mycobacterium* Species in Humans: Insights into Molecular Epidemiology, Virulence, and Antibiotic Resistance

Yi-Wen Liao, Yu-Rong Qin and Liang Wang

Abstract

Drug-resistant tuberculosis (TB) and non-tuberculous mycobacteria (NTM) infections pose significant global health challenges. Understanding the genomic diversity, pathogenicity, and mechanisms of antibiotic resistance in *Mycobacterium* species is critical for developing effective diagnostic tools and therapeutic strategies. This study conducted a comparative analysis of 632 *Mycobacterium* genomes obtained from the public database Bacterial and Viral Bioinformatics Resource Center (BV-BRC). The analysis focused on *Mycobacterium* tuberculosis (Mtb) and NTM. Techniques included comparative genome analysis, multilocus sequence typing (MLST), and phylogenetic analysis to identify sequence types (STs) and characterize virulence factors and antibiotic resistance genes. The study identified significant sequence types, with ST21 and ST27 being the most prevalent, associated with high transmission potential, virulence, and multidrug resistance. Analysis of virulence factors highlighted the essential roles of *ESX-1*, *ESX-3*, and *ESX-5* secretion systems in host immune evasion and nutrient acquisition. Antibiotic resistance profiles revealed the widespread presence of resistance genes, including those conferring resistance to aminoglycosides (e.g., *AAC(2′)-Ic*) and macrolides (e.g., *Erm(37)*). Efflux pump genes such as *efpA* and *mtrA* were prevalent, contributing significantly to multidrug resistance. These findings give insights into the genomic diversity and molecular mechanisms driving pathogenicity and drug resistance in *Mycobacterium* species. The results identify key targets for the development of innovative diagnostic tools and therapeutic interventions, advancing efforts to combat drug-resistant TB and NTM infections. Furthermore, this research underscores the importance of genomic surveillance in informing public health strategies to mitigate the spread of drug-resistant *Mycobacterium* strains.

Keywords: *Mycobacterium*, genomics, multilocus sequence typing (MLST), virulence factors, ESX secretion systems, antibiotic resistance

1. Introduction

1.1 Introduction to *Mycobacterium*

The genus *Mycobacterium*, part of the phylum Actinobacteria, comprises over 190 Gram-positive, non-motile, and aerobic species, many of which inhabit soil and water [1]. The most prominent member, *Mycobacterium tuberculosis* (Mtb), is the causative agent of tuberculosis (TB), a disease that has afflicted humans for centuries [2]. In addition to Mtb, other notable species include non-tuberculous mycobacteria (NTM), such as *Mycobacterium avium* and *Mycobacterium* intracellulare, which are opportunistic pathogens, particularly in immunocompromised individuals [3]. *Mycobacterium* species are characterized by their complex cell wall structures, rich in mycolic acids, conferring unique resistance to environmental stressors and antimicrobial agents [4]. This complexity makes them challenging to culture and treat, requiring specialized laboratory techniques. Advances in genomic technologies have enabled researchers to uncover the genomic features of various *Mycobacterium* strains, enhancing our understanding of their biology, pathogenic mechanisms, and antibiotic resistance.

1.2 Genomic characteristics of *Mycobacterium* species

M. tuberculosis, the primary pathogen responsible for tuberculosis, has a genome of approximately 4.4 mega-bases (Mb) and contains around 4000 genes [5]. A high GC content of 65% helps stabilize its genome under extreme conditions. The Mtb genome includes genes essential for cell wall synthesis, virulence factors, and antibiotic resistance mechanisms. Significant genetic variability within Mtb strains, especially across different geographical regions, offers important insights for epidemiological studies. In contrast, *M. canetti*, a close relative of Mtb with lower pathogenicity, has a genome size of approximately 4.5 Mb [6]. Although capable of causing tuberculosis, infections caused by *M. canetti* are relatively rare. Its genome contains unique genes that may be associated with its lower virulence, and these genes are currently under investigation. While M. *canetti* exhibits resistance to certain antibiotics, its resistance genes differ from those found in Mtb, suggesting novel therapeutic avenues. *M. avium*, commonly found in the environment and associated with birds and swine, has a larger genome of approximately 5.2 Mb [7]. This species contains diverse genes that enhance environmental adaptability and nutrient metabolism. *Mycobacterium intracellulare*, part of the *M. avium* complex (MAC), primarily causes pulmonary infections. Its genome is also around 6.5 Mb and is characterized by an abundance of metabolic genes that support its survival within host cells. *M. intracellulare* exhibits resistance to various antibiotics, particularly first-line anti-TB drugs, and effectively evades the host immune response, facilitating its proliferation in immunocompromised individuals [8].

1.3 Progress in genomic research of *Mycobacterium* species

Virulence refers to the ability of bacterial pathogens to cause disease, largely driven by specific virulence factors, which are characteristics or gene products that enhance the pathogen's ability to infect, survive, and proliferate within a host. These factors play critical roles in the pathogenicity of *Mycobacterium* species, which can be categorized into adherence, immune modulation, stress survival, effector delivery systems, and metabolic adaptation. Whole-genome sequencing (WGS) has made significant strides in uncovering *Mycobacterium* bacteria's virulence and drug resistance mechanisms, providing insights into the molecular basis of pathogenicity and resistance. The Virulence Factor Database (VFDB) provides a framework for understanding these mechanisms, classifying virulence factors based on their functions, such as adherence, biofilm formation, and immune evasion. Among *Mycobacterium* species, specialized effector delivery systems, particularly the ESX secretion systems, are vital for pathogenicity and immune evasion, with ESX-1, ESX-3, and ESX-5 receiving particular attention [9]. The ESX-1 system is closely associated with the bacterium's ability to invade host cells and evade immune responses. By secreting proteins like ESAT-6 and CFP-10, the ESX-1 system helps Mtb disrupt host cell membranes, facilitating successful infection and immune evasion [10]. ESX-3 plays a critical role in metal ion metabolism, particularly in acquiring iron and zinc, which is vital for the bacterium's survival [11]. ESX-5, predominantly studied in NTM, plays a significant role in host immune modulation and the establishment of chronic infections [12]. Genomic studies of these secretion systems have elucidated their central role in *Mycobacterium* virulence and have identified potential targets for the development of new anti-tuberculosis therapies. In addition to the ESX secretion systems, genomic studies have revealed other important virulence factors in *Mycobacterium*. Mycolic acids, for example, are essential components of the mycobacterial cell wall, conferring significant resistance to antibiotics and the host immune system. Through genomic analysis, researchers have gained a deeper understanding of the gene networks that regulate the synthesis of mycolic acids, offering new insights into the construction of the mycobacterial cell wall and its resistance mechanisms to drugs [5, 6].

The advancements in genomic research have also extended to NTMs, such as *M. avium* and *M. intracellulare*, where WGS has been used to uncover genetic determinants of resistance and adaptability. These species often carry genes that facilitate environmental persistence and opportunistic infections, with research highlighting the importance of metabolic flexibility in their ability to survive in diverse environments, including within host macrophages [13]. Identifying genes related to lipid metabolism, cell envelope synthesis, and immune evasion underscores the complexity of their pathogenicity and persistence.

Regarding antibiotic resistance, genomic studies have identified various gene mutations linked to drug resistance. The resistance of Mtb is primarily associated with mutations in genes that confer resistance to a range of antibiotics, including isoniazid (INH), rifampin (RIF), and fluoroquinolones (FQs). For example, mutations in the katG gene are associated with resistance to isoniazid, while mutations in the rpoB gene lead to rifampin resistance [14, 15]. These mutations alter the antibiotic's target or reduce its activity, allowing Mtb to evade the effects of the drugs. Furthermore, studies of multidrug-resistant tuberculosis (MDR-TB) and extensively drug-resistant tuberculosis (XDR-TB) strains have uncovered the cumulative effects of multiple gene mutations, revealing the global spread of these resistant strains through genomic analysis.

Comparative genomic analyses between drug-resistant and drug-sensitive strains have further advanced our understanding of resistance mechanisms. Studies have revealed that drug resistance in *Mycobacterium* species is not solely due to chromosomal mutations but also involves gene expression changes, efflux pumps, and biofilm formation, which collectively contribute to reduced drug susceptibility. Using transcriptomics and proteomics alongside WGS allows for a more comprehensive analysis of these mechanisms, providing a holistic view of how *Mycobacterium* adapts to antimicrobial pressure [16]. Beyond resistance, genomics has been instrumental in tracing the transmission and evolution of *Mycobacterium* strains. Phylogenetic studies have shown the global distribution of Mtb lineages and their association with specific resistance profiles. Genome-wide association studies (GWAS) have been used to identify genetic markers linked to virulence and resistance, providing a foundation for future diagnostic and therapeutic development [17].

Overall, genomic studies of *Mycobacterium* have greatly expanded our knowledge of their pathogenicity, resistance, and epidemiology. This study aims to analyze the genomic diversity, virulence factors, and antibiotic resistance mechanisms of *Mycobacterium* species, with a focus on leveraging these insights for therapeutic and diagnostic advancements. The application of genomic tools in clinical settings, such as WGS or SERS for rapid diagnosis and resistance profiling, is transforming the management of TB and NTM infections [18, 19]. Continued research into the genomic basis of virulence and resistance will be crucial for developing new strategies to combat these infections. As drug-resistant strains of Mtb and NTMs continue to pose a significant public health threat, integrating genomic data into drug development and public health surveillance will play a critical role in controlling the spread of these bacteria.

2. Methods for genomic analysis

This study acquired genomic data for *Mycobacterium* species from the BV-BRC website (https://www.bv-brc.org/). The selection criteria for the data included (a) host specificity to humans, (b) genome quality classified as "good," and (c) complete genome status. This rigorous filtering resulted in the download of 632 high-quality genomic sequences, which served as the foundation for our analyses. We utilized a Linux environment for phylogenetic analysis and employed the Roary software to perform pan-genome analysis [20]. Roary clustered gene families across the genomic datasets, allowing us to identify core and accessory genes within the samples. Subsequently, we constructed a phylogenetic tree based on the core genome, illustrating the *Mycobacterium* strains' evolutionary relationships. The constructed tree was visualized using the iTOL (https://itol.embl.de/) web platform, facilitating the clear depiction of phylogenetic relationships and genetic variations. To conduct multilocus sequence typing (MLST), we utilized the "mlst" software (https://pubmlst.org/multilocus-sequence-typing). We prepared genomic sequence files and employed mlst to extract specific core genes. These extracted sequences were compared against the MLST database to determine the MLST types for each strain. This analysis enabled us to characterize the epidemiological patterns of the *Mycobacterium* strains and identify those with similar genetic backgrounds. For the assessment of virulence and antibiotic resistance genes, we implemented Abricate software. We selected appropriate databases for targeted gene comparison, including the Virulence Factor Database (VFDB) and the Comprehensive Antibiotic Resistance Database (CARD). Abricate facilitated the identification of virulence and resistance genes present in our samples by cross-referencing them with the chosen databases, producing detailed analytical reports. In summary, our methodology incorporated various genomic tools to analyze *Mycobacterium* species' genomic features and epidemiological characteristics. The integration of Linux for phylogenetic analysis, Roary for tree construction, MLST for typing, and Abricate for virulence and resistance analysis enabled a comprehensive understanding of these bacteria's genetic diversity and evolutionary dynamics.

3. Results and discussion of molecular epidemiological genomic analyses of *Mycobacterium*: Genotyping and MLST analysis

The molecular epidemiology of *Mycobacterium* species, particularly *Mycobacterium tuberculosis* (Mtb), has become a pivotal area of research due to its implications in understanding transmission dynamics, antimicrobial resistance, and global disease control. With advancements in molecular techniques and genomics, researchers can now apply highly detailed analyses to track the spread of *Mycobacterium* strains, identify key genetic variations, and monitor resistance patterns. Implementing multilocus sequence typing (MLST) as a genotyping tool has significantly improved our ability to characterize *Mycobacterium* strains at a molecular level, particularly in conjunction with whole-genome sequencing (WGS). In this chapter, we will explore various molecular methods used in epidemiological studies of *Mycobacterium* and their common genotypes, focusing on MLST-based analysis and its role in revealing critical epidemiological patterns.

3.1 Common genotypes of *Mycobacterium*

The application of MLST in tuberculosis research has enabled the systematic classification and analysis of Mtb strains. For example, MLST can reveal strain transmission's geographic and epidemiological characteristics by comparing MLST profiles of different Mtb strains. MLST can efficiently type different *M. tuberculosis* strains by analyzing sequence variations in several conserved genes. MLST targets several core genes in *Mycobacterium* studies, such as S14Z, L35, S19, L19, S12, S8, L16, and S7. This high-resolution method is well-suited for tracking the transmission routes of different strains, thanks to its accuracy and reproducibility. Some common genotypes identified in molecular epidemiological studies include the Beijing genotype, which has been strongly associated with drug resistance, displaying resistance to multiple antibiotics. The global dissemination of the Beijing genotype is notable, with a widespread presence in East Asia and parts of Western countries, especially in highly urbanized areas. Another common genotype is the H37Rv strain, the first Mtb strain to be fully sequenced and remains widely used in laboratory research [21]. This strain is prevalent in Western Europe, particularly in countries like the Netherlands, where its spread is linked to regional epidemiological patterns and variable drug resistance profiles [22]. The West African 1/2 genotypes, commonly found in West Africa, are closely tied to the local epidemiology of tuberculosis, reflecting specific environmental and population factors in that region. Additionally, the Euro-American genotype is prevalent in Europe and the Americas, where its spread is influenced by specific geographic and social factors [23].

3.2 Analysis of common sequence types in *Mycobacterium* strains

In this study, we analyzed 632 *Mycobacterium* strains and identified that ST21 and ST27 were the most prevalent sequence types (STs), particularly in Mtb strains, shown in **Figure 1**. The high detection rate of these STs in clinical samples highlights their potential roles in host adaptation, virulence, and drug resistance. ST21 is considered an ancient sequence type, and studies suggest that this ST has strong transmission capabilities across various environments and hosts. The pathogenicity of ST21 strains is notably high, with specific mutation patterns linked to drug resistance. For example, ST21 strains are frequently associated with multidrug-resistant tuberculosis (MDR-TB), a finding corroborated by epidemiological studies in several countries [24, 25].

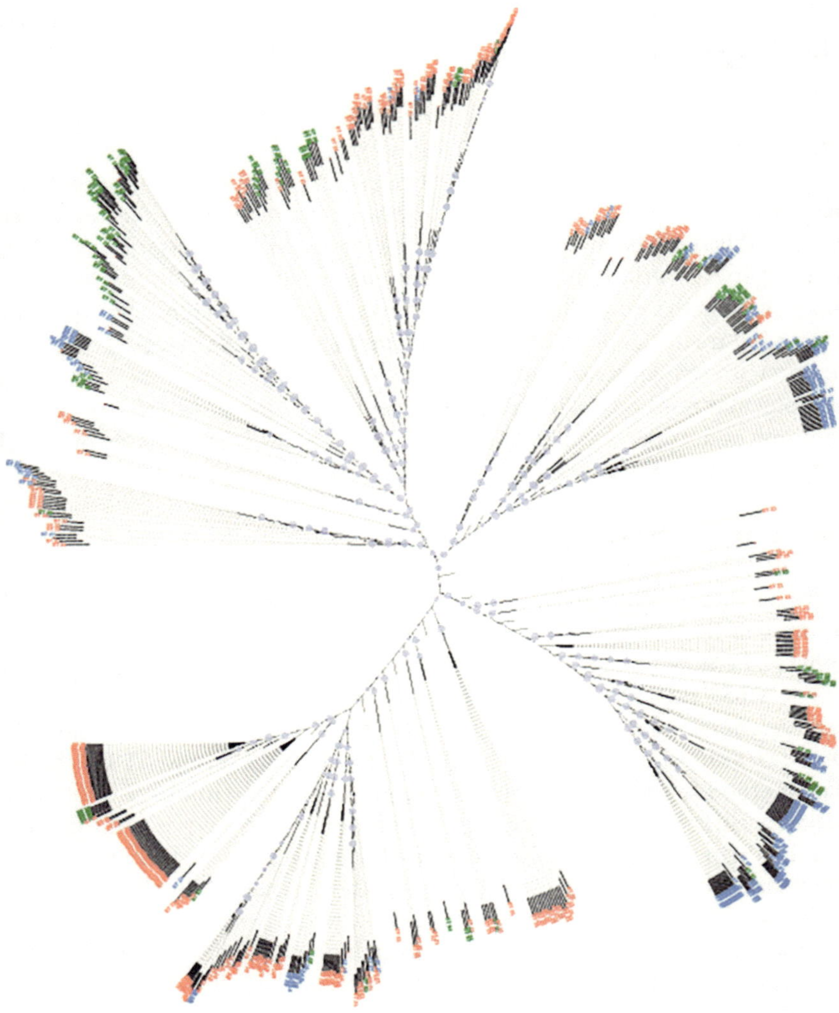

Figure 1.
Phylogeny and MLST distribution of Mycobacterium *strains. The innermost ring represents the types of* Mycobacteria, *with purple indicating the* Mycobacterium tuberculosis *complex (MTBC) and blue representing non-tuberculous mycobacteria (NTM). The outer ring denotes the MLST sequence types (STs) assigned to each strain.*

The widespread dissemination of ST21 can also be attributed to its distinct genetic background. Research indicates that ST21 strains often carry genes related to virulence and adaptability, which may enhance their ability to evade host immune responses and increase the success rate of infection. This makes ST21 an important target for further epidemiological surveillance and public health intervention. Similarly, ST27 strains also exhibit significant transmission potential and are distributed across various geographic regions. ST27 strains have notably increased infection rates in Europe and South America, particularly among immunosuppressed populations. The unique genomic structure of ST27 provides it with advantages in environmental adaptability. For instance, ST27 strains demonstrate varying antibiotic resistance, presenting new challenges to public health. The detection of resistance-related mutations in ST27 strains further underscores the importance of continued monitoring, as their spread may lead to the emergence of novel resistant lineages [26]. Other sequence types, such as ST32 and ST28, have been frequently reported in multiple studies and are linked to drug-resistant strains in certain regions. The widespread occurrence of these STs suggests that specific sequence types play critical roles in epidemiological monitoring and public health strategies. Apart from the four major STs, our analysis identified several other STs, including ST29, ST41, ST88, ST26, ST4, ST11, ST33, ST90, ST18, ST37, ST38, ST59, ST63, ST71, and ST84. While these STs were less prevalent in the overall analysis, they may have potential epidemiological significance in specific regions or populations. In particular, ST41 and ST88 were found to be more common in non-tuberculosis *Mycobacterium* (NTM) samples from certain clinical cases, reflecting their potential pathogenicity under specific pathological conditions [27, 28].

In conclusion, applying MLST in *Mycobacterium* genotyping and molecular epidemiology has revolutionized our understanding of strain diversity, transmission patterns, and resistance mechanisms. Identifying key STs, such as ST21 and ST27, and their roles in pathogenicity and drug resistance emphasizes the importance of ongoing surveillance and research. Understanding these strains' genomic and epidemiological characteristics will be vital in shaping effective public health strategies and improving the control of tuberculosis and other *Mycobacterium*-related diseases.

4. Results and discussion of virulence factors of the *Mycobacterium* genus

4.1 ESX secretion systems virulence

A key aspect of *Mycobacterium* virulence lies in its specialized secretion systems, notably the ESX family (Type VII secretion systems), which are essential for secreting effector proteins involved in pathogenesis, immune evasion, and intracellular survival. This study examines the presence and distribution of various virulence factors within the ESX family across 632 *Mycobacterium* strains, as shown in **Figure 2**.

4.1.1 Ecc proteins

The Ecc proteins (EccA1, EccA3, EccA5, EccB1, EccB3, EccB5, EccC3, EccCa1, EccCa5, EccCb1, EccCb5, EccD1, EccD3, EccD5, EccE1, EccE3, and EccE5) are structural and functional components of the ESX secretion systems. These proteins were detected in all 632 *Mycobacterium* strains, demonstrating their highly conserved and essential roles across various species. EccA proteins, as AAA+ ATPases, provide energy for protein secretion, a critical function for the ESX system's operation [29]. EccB and EccC proteins are integral membrane components, with EccC playing a pivotal role in substrate recognition and translocation [30]. The EccD protein forms the membrane channel through which effector proteins are secreted, while EccE stabilizes the secretion machinery. In this study, the presence of EccC3, EccCa5, EccCb5, EsxH, esxM, esxN, and the Rv1794 virulence genes was confirmed in all the analyzed strains, underscoring the functional integrity of the ESX secretion system across multiple *Mycobacterium* species.

4.1.2 Esp proteins

The Esp proteins (EspA, EspB, EspC, EspD, EspG3, and EspK) are the ESX-1 secretion system substrates and play critical roles in *Mycobacterium* virulence [31]. EspA is essential for the secretion of key virulence factors *EsxA* and *EsxB*, and

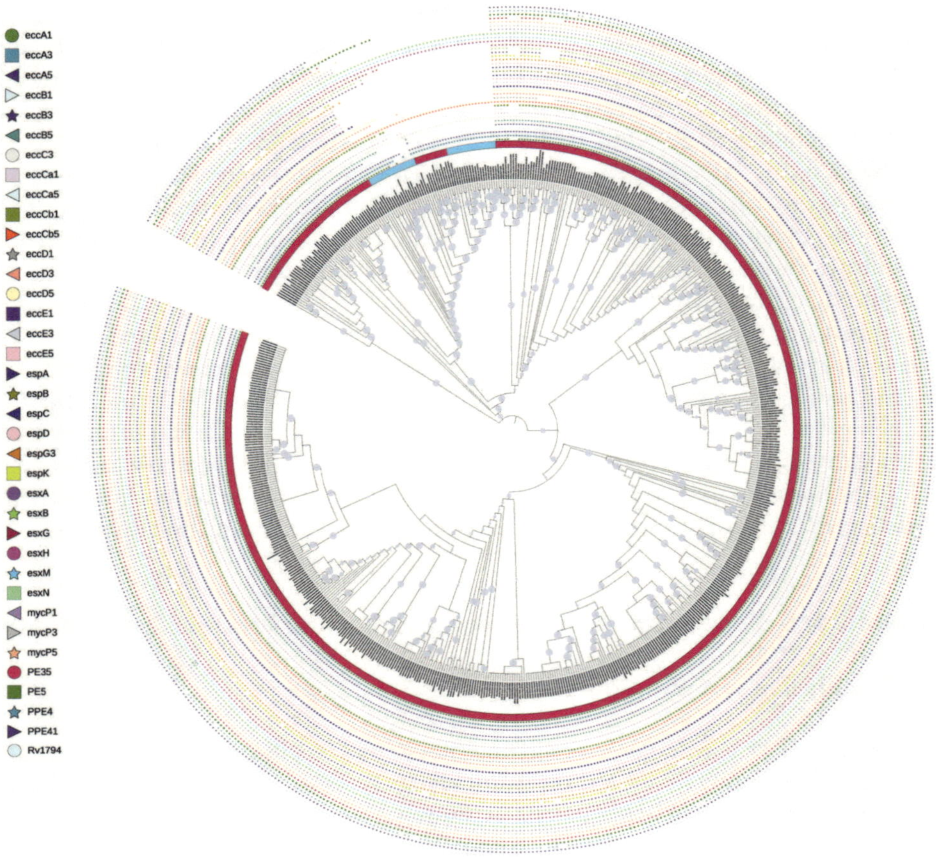

Figure 2.
Phylogeny of Mycobacterium *strains and ESX-related virulence genes from the VFDB database. The innermost ring represents the types of* Mycobacteria, *with purple indicating MTBC and blue representing NTM. The outer ring displays the presence (colored) or absence (uncolored) of 37 ESX-related virulence genes identified from the VFDB database for each strain.*

mutants lacking EspA are defective in this secretion, resulting in attenuated virulence. EspB, on the other hand, stabilizes the ESX-1 secretion machinery and modulates the host immune response by inhibiting antigen presentation, thereby facilitating immune evasion. EspC and EspD, though less well understood, contribute to the structural integrity of the secretion system. In contrast, EspG3, part of the ESX-3 system, is thought to be involved in metal ion acquisition, particularly iron and zinc. EspK may interact with host proteins to enhance bacterial survival within macrophages. The study revealed that Esp proteins (*EspA*, *EspB*, *EspC*, *EspD*, *EspG3*, and *EspK*) were only present in *M. tuberculosis*, *M. canettii*, *M. bovis*, *M. africanum*, *M. decipiens*, and *M. orygis*. At the same time, they were absent in other *Mycobacterium* species, indicating species-specific roles in virulence.

4.1.3 Esx proteins (EsxA, EsxB, EsxG, EsxH, EsxM, and EsxN)

Esx proteins, particularly *EsxA* (*ESAT-6*) and *EsxB* (*CFP-10*), are central to the virulence of *M. tuberculosis*. These small, secreted proteins form a heterodimer that disrupts the host cell membrane, allowing bacterial escape from host phagosomes [32].

EsxA and EsxB are highly immunogenic and are critical antigens in TB diagnostic tests. Other members of the Esx family, such as EsxG and EsxH, are involved in the bacterium's response to metal ion limitation. At the same time, EsxM and EsxN are less well-characterized but likely contribute to immune evasion. This study found *EsxH*, *EsxM*, and *EsxN* in all 632 *Mycobacterium* strains analyzed. However, EsxA and EsxB were missing in *M. avium*, *M. bovis*, *M. colombiense*, *M. heckeshornense*, *M. intracellulare*, *M. malmoense*, *M. paraintracellulare*, *M. shigaense*, *M. simiae*, *M. tuberculosis*, *M. ulcerans*, and *M. yongonense*, while EsxG was absent in *M. avium*, *M. colombiense*, *M. intracellulare*, *M. malmoense*, *M. paraintracellulare*, *M. simiae*, and *M. yongonense*, indicating variability in the presence of these proteins among different species.

4.1.4 Mycosin proteins

Mycosins (*MycP1*, *MycP3*, and *MycP5*) are proteases associated with the ESX secretion systems. MycP1, linked to the ESX-1 system, is crucial for the secretion of EsxA and EsxB by cleaving EspB, which aids in the assembly of the secretion machinery. MycP3 and MycP5, associated with the ESX-3 and ESX-5 systems, respectively, are believed to perform similar roles in processing and secreting effector proteins [33]. This study showed that MycP1, MycP3, and MycP5 were present in all *M. canettii*, *M. africanum*, *M. bovis*, *M. decipiens*, *M. kansasii*, *M. lacus*, *M. orygis*, *M. riyadhense*, and *M. shinjukuense* strains, and in the majority of *M. tuberculosis* strains (550/556). However, these proteins were absent in other *Mycobacterium* species, such as *M. avium*, *M. colombiense*, *M. gordonae*, *M. heckeshornense*, *M. intracellulare*, *M. malmoense*, *M. marinum*, *M. paraintracellulare*, *M. shigaense*, *M. simiae*, *M. ulcerans*, and *M. yongonense*, suggesting that these proteases may play species-specific roles in virulence and pathogenesis.

4.1.5 PE/PPE proteins

The proline-glutamate/proline-proline-glutamate (PE/PPE) protein families (PE35, PE5, PPE4, and PPE41) are unique to mycobacteria and are defined by their conserved proline-glutamate (PE) or proline-proline-glutamate (PPE) motifs [34]. The ESX-5 system often secretes these proteins and has been implicated in immune evasion. PE35 and PPE41 are key substrates of the ESX-1 system, with PE35 contributing to the stabilization of the secretion machinery and PPE41 playing a critical role in modulating the host immune response. Mutations in PPE41 have been associated with attenuated virulence in animal models [35]. This study detected PE35, PE5, PPE4, and PPE41 in 547 strains, including 522 *M. tuberculosis* strains, 23 *M. canettii* strains, one *M. africanum strain*, and one *M. orygis* strain. These proteins were absent in 37 strains, including *M. avium*, *M. colombiense*, *M. intracellulare*, *M. paraintracellulare*, *M. simiae*, and *M. yongonense*. The remaining strains contained at least one of the genes encoding these proteins, highlighting their variable presence among different species.

4.1.6 Rv1794

Rv1794 is a lesser-known protein associated with the ESX-1 secretion system. While its precise role in virulence remains unclear, it is believed to contribute to the stability and function of the ESX-1 machinery [36]. In this study, Rv1794 was detected in all 632 *Mycobacterium* strains analyzed, suggesting its widespread presence and potential importance across various species.

4.2 Non-ESX secretion systems virulence

Apart from the well-known ESX secretion systems involved in effector protein transport, we have conducted a thorough analysis of 29 additional virulence genes associated with *Mycobacterium* species, shown in **Figure 3**. These virulence factors belong to various categories: adherence, exotoxins, immune modulation, nutritional/metabolic factors, regulation, and stress survival. These diverse factors collectively contribute to the pathogen's ability to establish infection, persist in hostile environments, and evade the host immune response, each playing a critical role in the bacterium's pathogenicity.

4.2.1 Adherence

Adherence to host cells is the critical first step in any successful infection, enabling pathogens to anchor themselves to host tissues and resist removal by fluid flow. This allows bacteria to colonize host tissues and establish a stable infection. In *Mycobacterium*, adherence factors mediate the interaction between the bacterium and host cells, especially macrophages, facilitating entry and colonization. The *fbpA*,

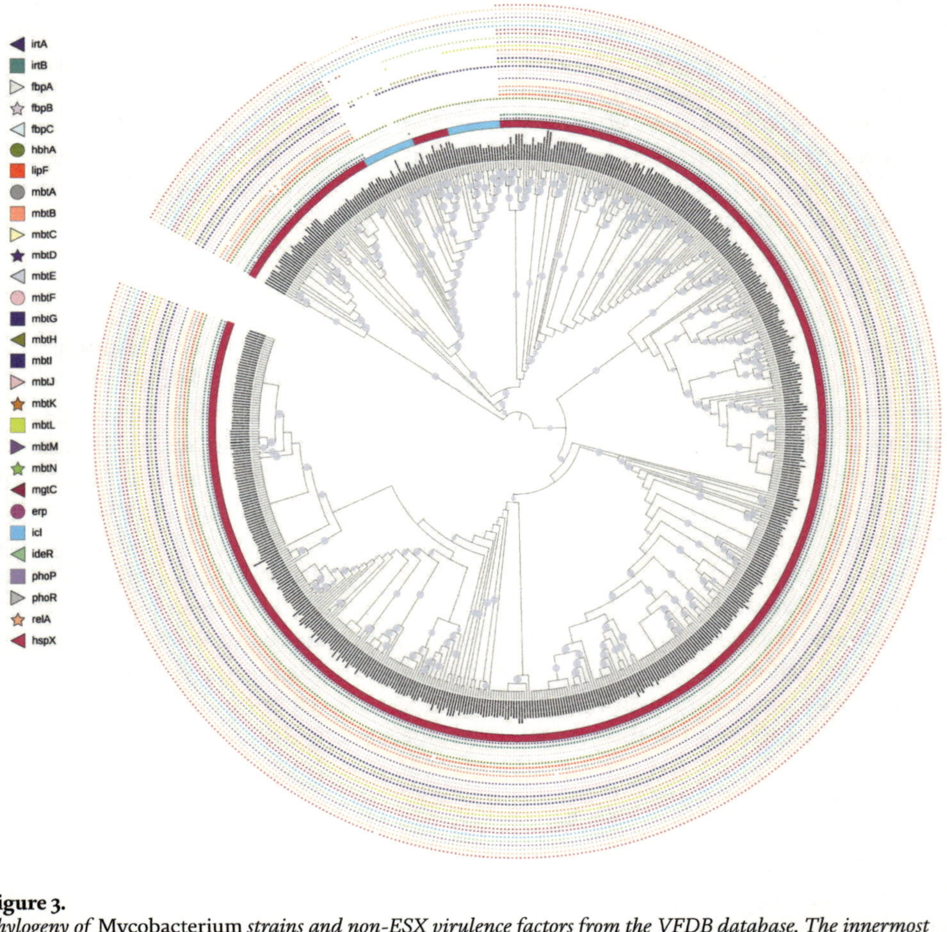

Figure 3.
Phylogeny of Mycobacterium *strains and non-ESX virulence factors from the VFDB database. The innermost ring represents the types of Mycobacteria, with purple indicating MTBC and blue representing NTM. The outer ring marks the presence (colored) or absence (uncolored) of 29 non-ESX virulence factors identified from the VFDB database for each strain.*

fbpB, and *fbpC* genes in *Mycobacterium* tuberculosis encode fibronectin-binding proteins (FbpA, FbpB, and FbpC) that form the antigen 85 complex, crucial for bacterial adhesion to fibronectin, aiding in colonization, cell wall integrity, and immune evasion during infection [37]. In our study of 632 *Mycobacterium* genomes, the *fbpA*, *fbpB*, and *fbpC* genes were present in nearly all *Mycobacterium* strains, indicating their fundamental role in adhesion across different species. Interestingly, the only exceptions were *M. heckeshornense* and *M. shigaense*, which lacked the *fbpB* gene. The Heparin-Binding Hemagglutinin Adhesin (HbhA) protein, encoded by the *hbhA* gene, is essential for *M. tuberculosis* adhesion to epithelial cells and macrophages, promoting colonization and systemic infection. Genome analysis shows that *hbhA* is present in nearly all *Mycobacterium* strains except *M. heckeshornense*, underscoring its widespread role in pathogenicity.

4.2.2 Exotoxins

Exotoxins are potent virulence factors in *Mycobacterium* that damage host cells and modulate immune responses, allowing the bacterium to evade defenses and persist within the host. One exotoxin-related gene, *lipF*, encodes a probable esterase/lipase that breaks down host lipid molecules into fatty acids, which serve as a vital carbon source during infection, particularly in nutrient-limited conditions [37]. This ability to exploit host lipid reserves for survival is critical for *Mycobacterium*'s long-term persistence, and our study consistently found the *lipF* gene in *M. tuberculosis*, *M. canettii*, *M. africanum*, *M. bovis*, *M. decipiens*, and *M. orygis*.

4.2.3 Nutritional/metabolic factors

In *Mycobacterium*, nutritional and metabolic virulence factors are crucial for extracting essential nutrients like iron and magnesium from the host, allowing the bacterium to thrive in nutrient-poor environments during infection. The *irtA* and *irtB* genes encode ABC transporter proteins involved in iron acquisition, a critical process for bacterial survival, particularly under the iron-limited conditions imposed by the host immune system [38]. These genes, detected in *M. tuberculosis*, *M. canettii*, *M. bovis*, *M. africanum*, *M. decipiens*, and *M. orygis*, but absent in other *Mycobacterium* species, highlight the importance of iron acquisition in these pathogens. Additionally, *mgtC* encodes a protein essential for magnesium acquisition, particularly in low-magnesium environments like macrophages, where it supports bacterial survival. Mutants lacking *mgtC* show reduced survival, emphasizing its role in pathogenesis. The widespread presence of *mgtC* in pathogenic strains underlines its significance in adapting to host-imposed nutrient stress conditions.

4.2.4 Immune modulation

In *Mycobacterium*, several virulence factors contribute to immune modulation by either dampening or subverting the host's immune defenses. The *ideR* gene encodes a transcriptional regulator that controls genes involved in iron homeostasis and oxidative stress response, helping bacteria survive immune-induced oxidative stress while indirectly affecting immune cell activation through iron regulation [39]. Our study found *ideR* present in all pathogenic *Mycobacterium* species, underscoring its role in immune evasion. The *relA* gene, responsible for the stringent response, helps bacteria conserve resources during nutrient limitation and stress, enhancing persistence during immune challenges. *relA* was detected in all *Mycobacterium* strains, highlighting its critical role in survival during host-imposed stress [40].

4.2.5 Stress survival

In *Mycobacterium*, several genes enhance bacterial survival under host-induced stresses such as acidic pH, oxidative stress, and nutrient deprivation, contributing to persistent infections. The *hspX* gene encodes a heat shock protein that helps the bacterium withstand oxidative and heat stress by stabilizing proteins, ensuring survival in hostile environments [41]. HspX was found in all pathogenic *Mycobacterium* strains, highlighting its role in stress survival. The *phoP* gene, a transcriptional regulator, enables bacterial adaptation to acidic conditions within macrophages, and mutants lacking *phoP* exhibit reduced virulence [42]. Our analysis confirmed *phoP* in nearly all *Mycobacterium* strains, emphasizing its role in stress survival and virulence.

4.2.6 Regulation

In *Mycobacterium*, regulatory factors control gene expression in response to external stimuli, enabling adaptation to various conditions. The *dosR* gene encodes a transcriptional regulator critical for the dormancy response, activating genes that allow the bacterium to enter a dormant state under hypoxia or nutrient limitation [43]. This dormancy is key for long-term survival and the persistence of latent infections. Our analysis found *dosR* in all pathogenic *Mycobacterium* strains, underscoring its role in chronic infection development.

5. Results and discussion of antibiotic resistance of *Mycobacterium* based on genomic analysis

In our comprehensive analysis of 632 *Mycobacterium* strains using the Comprehensive Antibiotic Resistance Database (CARD), several key resistance genes were identified, as shown in **Figure 4**. Among these, the aminoglycoside resistance gene AAC(2′)-Ic, which encodes an aminoglycoside acetyltransferase, was detected in 596 out of the 632 strains. This enzyme modifies aminoglycosides, rendering them ineffective against the bacterium, as shown in **Table 1**. The high prevalence of this gene underscores a significant resistance mechanism against aminoglycosides, suggesting that alternative treatments or combination therapies are necessary to bypass this resistance. For instance, using non-aminoglycoside antibiotics in combination with inhibitors that target the activity of AAC(2′)-Ic could be explored as a potential therapeutic strategy [44]. Regarding macrolide resistance, the erm(37) gene, which encodes a methyltransferase responsible for methylating 23S rRNA and preventing macrolide binding, was found in 563 strains. The widespread detection of erm(37) signifies a major challenge in using macrolides for treating *Mycobacterium* infections, particularly in tuberculosis (TB) management [45].

One of the most critical findings in our analysis was the detection of RbpA in all 632 strains. RbpA encodes an RNA polymerase-binding protein that modulates the function of RNA polymerase, a key enzyme targeted by rifampicin [46]. The presence of RbpA across all strains suggests that this protein plays a fundamental role in resistance to rifampicin, one of the cornerstone drugs in TB treatment [47]. The study also revealed mutations in rpoB, the gene encoding the β-subunit of RNA polymerase,

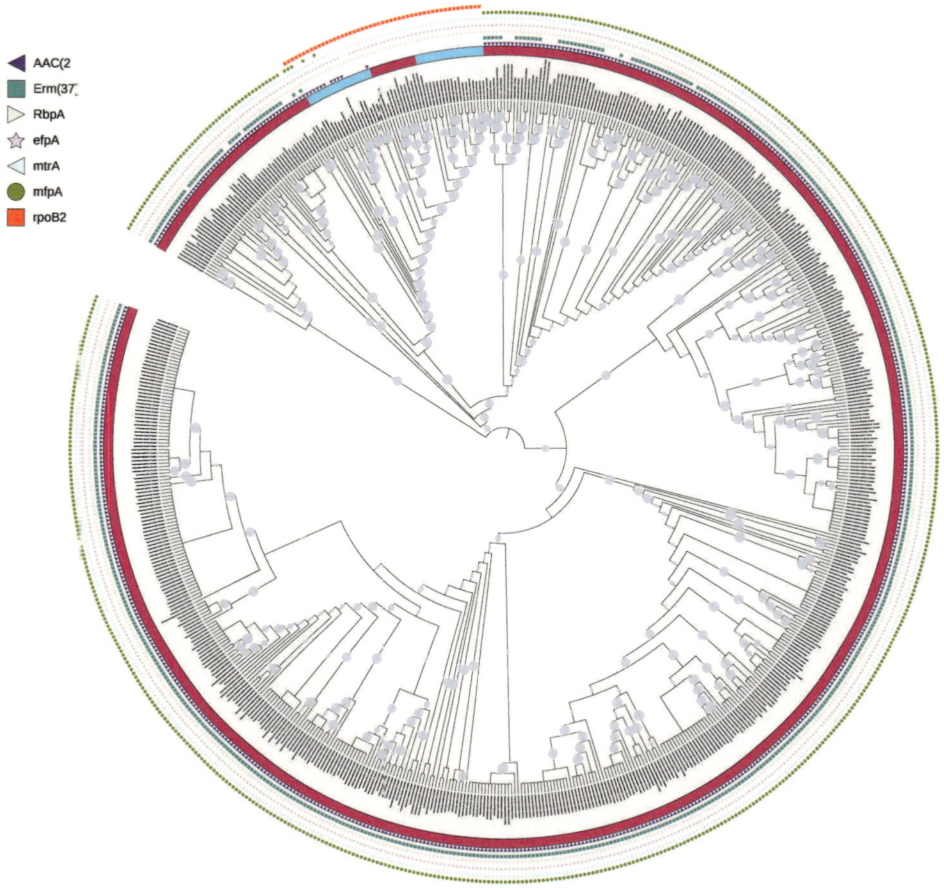

Figure 4.
Phylogeny of Mycobacterium *strains and antimicrobial resistance gene analysis. The innermost ring represents the types of* Mycobacteria, *with purple indicating MTBC and blue representing NTM. The outer ring shows the distribution of seven antimicrobial resistance genes identified from the CARD database, with a gene indicated by a colored segment and the absence indicated by an uncolored segment.*

a well-known mechanism of rifampicin resistance. Mutations in rpoB were present in most strains, while rpoB2, a homolog of rpoB, was detected in 49 strains. The presence of rpoB2 in a subset of the strains suggests that alternative pathways may also contribute to rifampicin resistance, adding complexity to the resistance profile of these bacteria. The combined detection of RbpA and rpoB mutations highlights the challenges of overcoming rifampicin resistance. It underscores the need for new drugs that effectively target RNA polymerase in resistant strains.

Efflux pump mechanisms were another significant area of resistance identified in our study. The gene efpA, which encodes a multidrug efflux pump that expels various antibiotics from the bacterial cell, was found in 631 strains. This efflux system allows the bacteria to survive in the presence of a wide range of antibiotics by reducing the intracellular concentration of the drugs, thereby decreasing their efficacy [48]. The high prevalence of efpA suggests that efflux mechanisms are a common strategy employed by *Mycobacterium* to resist treatment. Similarly, mtrA, another efflux-related gene, was detected in 630 strains. This gene is believed to play a role in bacterial survival under antibiotic pressure, although its exact mechanism in resistance

Gene	Product	Resistance	Proportion
AAC (2′)-Ic	AAC(2′)-Ic is a chromosomal-encoded aminoglycoside acetyltransferase in M. tuberculosis and *Mycobacterium* tuberculosis variant bovis.	Aminoglycoside	596/632
Erm (37)	Erm(37) is found in *Mycobacterium* species and confers the MLSb phenotype. In addition to methylation of A2058 this Erm methylates adjacent adenosines (A2057 and A2059) as well.	Lincosamide; macrolide; streptogramin	563/632
RbpA	RNA polymerase binding protein which confers resistance to rifampin.	Rifamycin	632/632
efpA	efpA is an MFS transporter found in *Mycobacterium tuberculosis*.	Isoniazid; rifamycin	631/632
mfpA	mfpA is a qnr homolog and a pentapeptide repeat protein that confers resistance to fluoroquinolones in *Mycolicibacterium smegmatis.*	Fluoroquinolone	631/632
mtrA	MtrA is a transcriptional activator of the MtrCDE multidrug efflux pump of *Neisseria gonorrhoeae*.	Macrolide; penam	630/632
rpoB2	Expression of the RNA polymerase (rpoB2) variant results in replacement of rifampin sensitivity with rifampin resistance.	Rifamycin	49/632

Table 1.
Summary of Antibiotic Resistance Genes in Mycobacterium *Strains Identified through CARD Database Analysis.*

needs further investigation. Targeting efflux pumps, possibly with specific inhibitors, could improve the retention and efficacy of conventional antibiotics, offering a promising avenue for enhancing treatment outcomes in multidrug-resistant TB.

Fluoroquinolone resistance, mediated by mfpA, was observed in 631 out of 632 strains. MfpA is a DNA mimic protein that protects DNA gyrase from fluoroquinolones, a class of antibiotics that target this enzyme [49]. The near-ubiquitous presence of mfpA in these strains indicates that fluoroquinolone resistance is widespread, further complicating treatment strategies [50]. Given the critical role of fluoroquinolones in TB therapy, particularly in drug-resistant cases, understanding the function of mfpA and developing strategies to counter its protective effect on DNA gyrase is essential.

The CARD database provided crucial insights into Mycobacterium resistance mechanisms; however, potential limitations should be acknowledged. The database relies on publicly available genomic data, which may exhibit geographic and sampling biases, potentially underrepresenting certain strains or resistance profiles. Additionally, while CARD effectively identified key resistance genes like AAC(2′)-Ic, erm(37), and mfpA, in silico predictions may not fully reflect their expression or functional relevance under clinical conditions. For example, genes like mtrA require further investigation to confirm their role in resistance. Addressing these limitations through experimental validation and incorporating more diverse genomic datasets will enhance the accuracy of resistance profiling.

In summary, our CARD-based comparative genomic analysis revealed a complex landscape of antibiotic resistance in *Mycobacterium* strains. Key genes such as AAC(2′)-Ic, erm(37), RbpA, rpoB, efpA, mtrA, and mfpA contribute to resistance against multiple drug classes, including aminoglycosides, macrolides, rifampicin, and fluoroquinolones. These findings emphasize the need for novel therapeutic approaches targeting these resistance mechanisms, including efflux pump inhibitors and new drugs that bypass the protective roles of RbpA and mfpA. Addressing these resistance factors is critical for improving the efficacy of current treatments and combating the growing threat of drug-resistant tuberculosis.

6. Limitations in this study

A key limitation of this study is its reliance on publicly available genomic data from the Bacterial and Viral Bioinformatics Resource Center (BV-BRC). While this database provides an extensive collection of Mycobacterium genomes, the dataset may be subject to incomplete or uneven sampling, which could introduce bias in the results. For example, certain geographic regions or clinical contexts may be underrepresented, limiting the generalizability of findings to the global population. Additionally, the quality of metadata associated with these genomes varies, and incomplete information on strain origin, clinical phenotype, or antibiotic susceptibility profiles can constrain the interpretation of results. Furthermore, reliance on computational analyses, such as multilocus sequence typing and phylogenetic reconstruction, may overlook nuances in phenotypic behavior and gene expression that experimental validation could address. Future studies incorporating well-curated datasets with detailed clinical metadata and integrating laboratory-based validation will be critical for overcoming these limitations and enhancing the robustness of the findings.

7. Summary and future directions

This study comprehensively analyzes key virulence factors and antibiotic resistance genes in 632 *Mycobacterium* strains, emphasizing the molecular features that contribute to pathogenicity and drug resistance. In terms of virulence, both ESX and non-ESX secretion systems were identified as critical in mediating *Mycobacterium* infections. Core proteins such as Ecc and Rv1794 were conserved across all strains. This finding highlights their essential role in bacterial survival and pathogenicity. These proteins involve various processes, including immune modulation, adherence, nutrient acquisition, and stress survival. However, proteins such as Esp, Esx, and the PE/PPE family showed variability among different strains, suggesting species-specific adaptations that may affect virulence and immune evasion strategies. This variability points to the evolutionary complexity of *Mycobacterium* species and their ability to adapt to various environmental and host challenges, which in turn influences their capacity to cause disease. Understanding these mechanisms is crucial for designing targeted therapies that can interfere with *Mycobacterium*'s infection processes. In addition to virulence factors, our study identified multiple antibiotic resistance genes, offering important insights into the molecular basis of resistance in *Mycobacterium* strains. Genes such as AAC(2′)-Ic, Erm(37), RbpA, efpA, mfpA, mtrA, and rpoB2 were detected with varying frequencies, demonstrating the widespread nature of resistance mechanisms across these strains. The findings from this study have significant implications for practical applications. For example, the identification of conserved core proteins, such as Ecc and Rv1794, offers potential targets for developing broad-spectrum vaccines effective against diverse *Mycobacterium* strains. Similarly, understanding the molecular basis of drug resistance can inform the design of rapid diagnostic tools to detect resistance genes, enabling timely and personalized treatment strategies. These advancements could enhance public health efforts to control the spread of drug-resistant *Mycobacterium* infections.

Declaration of competing interest

The authors declare that they have no known competing financial interests or personal relationships that could have appeared to influence the work reported in this paper.

Author details

Yi-Wen Liao*, Yu-Rong Qin and Liang Wang
Guangdong Provincial People's Hospital (Guangdong Academy of Medical Sciences), Southern Medical University, Guangzhou, China

*Address all correspondence to: lyw3706634@163.com

References

[1] Pai M, Kasaeva T, Swaminathan S. Covid-19's devastating effect on tuberculosis care - a path to recovery. The New England Journal of Medicine. 2022;**386**(16):1490-1493. DOI: 10.1056/NEJMp2118145

[2] Bagcchi S. WHO's global tuberculosis report 2022. Lancet Microbe. 2023;**4**(1):e20. DOI: 10.1016/S2666-5247(22)00359-7

[3] Dartois V, Dick T. Therapeutic developments for tuberculosis and nontuberculous mycobacterial lung disease. Nature Reviews. Drug Discovery. 2024;**23**(5):381-403. DOI: 10.1038/s41573-024-00897-5

[4] Takayama K, Wang C, Besra GS. Pathway to synthesis and processing of mycolic acids in *Mycobacterium tuberculosis*. Clinical Microbiology Reviews. 2005;**18**(1):81-101. DOI: 10.1128/CMR.18.1.81-101.2005

[5] Cole ST, Brosch R, Parkhill J, et al. Deciphering the biology of *Mycobacterium tuberculosis* from the complete genome sequence. Nature. 1998;**393**(6685):537-544. DOI: 10.1038/31159

[6] Supply P, Marceau M, Mangenot S, et al. Genomic analysis of smooth tubercle bacilli provides insights into ancestry and pathoadaptation of *Mycobacterium* tuberculosis. Nature Genetics. 2013;**45**(2):172-179. DOI: 10.1038/ng.2517

[7] Hidi L, Kovács GI, Szabó D, et al. Human blood vessel microbiota in healthy adults based on common femoral arteries of brain-dead multi-organ donors. Frontiers in Cellular and Infection Microbiology. 2022;**12**:1056319

[8] Kim BJ, Choi BS, Lim JS, et al. Complete genome sequence of *Mycobacterium* intracellulare strain ATCC 13950(T). Journal of Bacteriology. 2012;**194**(10):2750. DOI: 10.1128/JB.00295-12

[9] Toniolo C, Dhar N, McKinney JD. Uptake-independent killing of macrophages by extracellular *Mycobacterium* tuberculosis aggregates. The EMBO Journal. 2023;**42**(9):e113490. DOI: 10.15252/embj.2023113490

[10] Gries R, Chhen J, van Gumpel E, et al. Discovery of dual-active ethionamide boosters inhibiting the *Mycobacterium* tuberculosis ESX-1 secretion system. Cell Chemical Biology. 2024;**31**(4):699-711.e6. DOI: 10.1016/j.chembiol.2023.12.007

[11] Li B, He S, Tan Z, et al. Impaired ESX-3 induces Bedaquiline persistence in *Mycobacterium* abscessus growing under iron-limited conditions. Small Methods. 2023;**7**(9):e2300183

[12] Beckham KS, Ciccarelli L, Bunduc CM, et al. Structure of the mycobacterial ESX-5 type VII secretion system membrane complex by single-particle analysis. Nature Microbiology. 2017;**2**:17047

[13] Badia-Bringué G, Canive M, Vázquez P, et al. Genome-wide association study reveals quantitative trait loci and candidate genes associated with high interferon-gamma production in Holstein cattle naturally infected with *mMycobacterium bovis*. International Journal of Molecular Sciences. 2024;**25**(11):6165

[14] Li YF, Kong XL, Song WM, et al. Genomic analysis of lineage-specific

transmission of multidrug resistance tuberculosis in China. Emerging Microbes & Infections. 2024;**13**(1):2294858

[15] Comas I, Borrell S, Roetzer A, et al. Whole-genome sequencing of rifampicin-resistant *Mycobacterium tuberculosis* strains identifies compensatory mutations in RNA polymerase genes. Nature Genetics. 2011;**44**(1):106-110

[16] Cohen KA, Manson AL, Desjardins CA, Abeel T, Earl AM. Deciphering drug resistance in *Mycobacterium tuberculosis* using whole-genome sequencing: Progress, promise, and challenges. Genome Medicine. 2019;**11**(1):45

[17] Asner SA, Morré SA, Bochud PY, Greub G. Host factors and genetic susceptibility to infections due to intracellular bacteria and fastidious organisms. Clinical Microbiology and Infection. 2014;**20**(12):1246-1253. DOI: 10.1111/1469-0691.12806

[18] Xiong XS, Zhang XD, Yan JW, et al. Identification of *Mycobacterium tuberculosis* resistance to common antibiotics: An overview of current methods and techniques. Infection and Drug Resistance. 2024;**17**:1491-1506

[19] Wang L, Zhang XD, Tang JW, et al. Machine learning analysis of SERS fingerprinting for the rapid determination of *Mycobacterium tuberculosis* infection and drug resistance. Computational and Structural Biotechnology Journal. 2022;**20**:5364-5377

[20] Page AJ, Cummins CA, Hunt M, et al. Roary: Rapid large-scale prokaryote pan genome analysis. Bioinformatics. 2015;**31**(22):3691-3693

[21] Cole ST. Learning from the genome sequence of *Mycobacterium tuberculosis* H37Rv. FEBS Letters. 1999;**452**(1-2):7-10

[22] Conceição EC, Loubser J, Guimarães AEDS, et al. A genome-focused investigation reveals the emergence of a *Mycobacterium tuberculosis* strain related to multidrug-resistant tuberculosis in the Amazon region of Brazil. Microorganisms. 2024;**12**(9):1817

[23] Bruijnesteijn van Coppenraet LE, Savelkoul PH, Buffing N, et al. Amplified fragment length polymorphism analysis of human clinical isolates of *Mycobacterium haemophilum* from different continents. Clinical Microbiology and Infection. 2009;**15**(10):924-930

[24] Walker TM, Miotto P, Köser CU, et al. The 2021 WHO catalogue of *Mycobacterium tuberculosis* complex mutations associated with drug resistance: A genotypic analysis. Lancet Microbe. 2022;**3**(4):e265-e273

[25] Stavrum R, PrayGod G, Range N, et al. Increased level of acute phase reactants in patients infected with modern *Mycobacterium tuberculosis* genotypes in Mwanza, Tanzania. BMC Infectious Diseases. 2014;**14**:309

[26] Whatmore AM, Dawson C, Muchowski J, et al. Characterisation of north American Brucella isolates from marine mammals. PLoS One. 2017;**12**(9):e0184758

[27] Valcheva V, Mokrousov I, Rastogi N, Narvskaya O, Markova N. Molecular characterization of *Mycobacterium* tuberculosis isolates from different regions of Bulgaria. Journal of Clinical Microbiology. 2008;**46**(3):1014-1018

[28] Zozio T, Allix C, Gunal S, et al. Genotyping of *Mycobacterium* tuberculosis clinical isolates in two cities of Turkey: Description of a new family of genotypes that is phylogeographically specific for Asia Minor. BMC Microbiology. 2005;**5**:44

[29] Kriel NL, Newton-Foot M, Bennion OT, et al. Localization of EccA3 at the growing pole in *Mycobacterium smegmatis*. BMC Microbiology. 2022;**22**(1):140

[30] Bunduc CM, Fahrenkamp D, Wald J, et al. Structure and dynamics of a mycobacterial type VII secretion system. Nature. 2021;**593**(7859):445-448

[31] Wang Y, Tang Y, Lin C, et al. Crosstalk between the ancestral type VII secretion system ESX-4 and other T7SS in *Mycobacterium marinum*. iScience. 2021;**25**(1):103585

[32] Bao Y, Wang L, Sun J. Post-translational knockdown and post-secretional modification of EsxA determine contribution of EsxA membrane permeabilizing activity for mycobacterial intracellular survival. Virulence. 2021;**12**(1):312-328

[33] Sun D, Liu Q, He Y, et al. The putative propeptide of MycP1 in mycobacterial type VII secretion system does not inhibit protease activity but improves protein stability. Protein & Cell. 2013;**4**(12):921-931

[34] Priyanka SS, Varma-Basil M, Sharma M. C-terminal region of Rv1039c (PPE15) protein of *Mycobacterium tuberculosis* targets host mitochondria to induce macrophage apoptosis. Apoptosis. 2024;**29**(9-10):1757-1779

[35] Guo F, Wei J, Song Y, et al. Immunological effects of the PE/PPE family proteins of *Mycobacterium tuberculosis* and related vaccines. Frontiers in Immunology. 2023;**14**:1255920

[36] Bottai D, Di Luca M, Majlessi L, et al. Disruption of the ESX-5 system of *Mycobacterium tuberculosis* causes loss of PPE protein secretion, reduction of cell wall integrity and strong attenuation. Molecular Microbiology. 2012;**83**(6):1195-1209

[37] Copenhaver RH, Sepulveda E, Armitige LY, et al. A mutant of *Mycobacterium tuberculosis* H37Rv that lacks expression of antigen 85A is attenuated in mice but retains vaccinogenic potential. Infection and Immunity. 2004;**72**(12):7084-7095

[38] Arriaga-Guerrero AL, Hernández-Luna CE, Rigal-Leal J, et al. LipF increases rifampicin and streptomycin sensitivity in a *Mycobacterium tuberculosis* surrogate. BMC Microbiology. 2020;**20**(1):132

[39] Marcos-Torres FJ, Maurer D, Juniar L, Griese JJ. The bacterial iron sensor IdeR recognizes its DNA targets by indirect readout. Nucleic Acids Research. 2021;**49**(17):10120-10135

[40] Dahl JL, Kraus CN, Boshoff HI, et al. The role of RelMtb-mediated adaptation to stationary phase in long-term persistence of *Mycobacterium tuberculosis* in mice. Proceedings of the National Academy of Sciences of the United States of America. 2003;**100**(17):10026-10031. DOI: 10.1073/pnas.1631248100

[41] Zhou F, Xu X, Cui X, Pan W. Development and evaluation of a fusion polyprotein based on HspX and other antigen sequences for the serodiagnosis of tuberculosis. Frontiers in Immunology. 2021;**12**:726920

[42] Ahn SK, Tran V, Leung A, Ng M, Li M, Liu J. Recombinant

BCG overexpressing phoP-phoR confers enhanced protection against tuberculosis. Molecular Therapy. 2018;**26**(12):2863-2874

[43] Bucşan AN, Veatch A, Singh DK, et al. Response to hypoxia and the ensuing dysregulation of inflammation impacts *Mycobacterium* tuberculosis pathogenicity [published correction appears in Am J Respir Crit Care Med. 2022 Dec 1;206(11):1434. DOI: 10.1164/rccm.v206erratum12]. American Journal of Respiratory and Critical Care Medicine. 2022;**206**(1):94-104

[44] Paradise MR, Cook G, Poole RK, Rather PN. Mutations in aarE, the ubiA homolog of *Providencia stuartii*, result in high-level aminoglycoside resistance and reduced expression of the chromosomal aminoglycoside 2'-N-acetyltransferase. Antimicrobial Agents and Chemotherapy. 1998;**42**(4):959-962. DOI: 10.1128/AAC.42.4.959

[45] Andini N, Nash KA. Intrinsic macrolide resistance of the *Mycobacterium* tuberculosis complex is inducible. Antimicrobial Agents and Chemotherapy. 2006;**50**(7):2560-2562. DOI: 10.1128/AAC.00264-06

[46] Sudalaiyadum Perumal A, Vishwakarma RK, Hu Y, Morichaud Z, Brodolin K. RbpA relaxes promoter selectivity of *M. tuberculosis* RNA polymerase. Nucleic Acids Research. 2018;**46**(19):10106-10118. DOI: 10.1093/nar/gky714

[47] Jensen D, Manzano AR, Rammohan J, Stallings CL, Galburt EA. CarD and RbpA modify the kinetics of initial transcription and slow promoter escape of the *Mycobacterium tuberculosis* RNA polymerase. Nucleic Acids Research. 2019;**47**(13):6685-6698

[48] Wang S, Wang K, Song K, et al. Structures of the *Mycobacterium tuberculosis* efflux pump EfpA reveal the mechanisms of transport and inhibition. Nature Communications. 2024;**15**(1):7710

[49] Hegde SS, Vetting MW, Roderick SL, et al. A fluoroquinolone resistance protein from *Mycobacterium tuberculosis* that mimics DNA. Science. 2005;**308**(5727):1480-1483

[50] Ferber D. Biochemistry. Protein that mimics DNA helps tuberculosis bacteria resist antibiotics. Science. 2005;**308**(5727):1393

Chapter 2

The Prevalence, Risk Factors, and Drug Resistance Profiles of *Mycobacterium tuberculosis* in China: A Mini-Review

Xue-Song Xiong, Qin-Hui Zhu, Zhan-Zhong Liu, Ting-Ting Huang, Jin-Bin Fan, Xiao Zhao, Jian-Song Gu and Fen Li

Abstract

Mycobacterial infections are a group of infectious diseases caused by bacterial pathogens in the genus *Mycobacterium*, including *Mycobacterium tuberculosis* (MTB) complex, nontuberculous mycobacteria (NTM), and *Mycobacterium leprae*. Tuberculosis caused by *M. tuberculosis* has become the leading cause of death of a single infectious disease after novel coronavirus pneumonia. Over 90% of the pathogenic bacteria of human pulmonary tuberculosis are caused by MTB. The main transmission routes of MTB are airborne droplets and person-to-person contact, and it is easy to form an explosive epidemic due to its high contagion. Although the detection capacity of MTB in clinical laboratories has been dramatically improved, multidrug-resistant *M. tuberculosis* (MDR-TB) is an essential cause of tuberculosis treatment failure. It is attributed to the long treatment cycle and high health care costs, resulting in a substantial social and economic burden. China has been one of the highest burden countries with MDR-TB infections in the world. Therefore, the up-to-date data about the prevalence, risk factors, and antibiotic resistance profiles of MTB in China is of great significance for the effective control of the highly contagious bacterial pathogen in the country. In this mini-review, we went through the latest literature about the current infection rates, common risk factors for the infection, and the profiles of MTB resistance to common antibiotics, aiming to provide an overview of MTB infection in China and facilitate the control and eradication of the bacterial pathogen in the near future.

Keywords: tuberculosis, *Mycobacterium tuberculosis*, prevalence, risk factors, multidrug resistance profiles

1. Introduction

Tuberculosis (TB), caused by the ancient bacterial pathogen *Mycobacterium tuberculosis* (MTB), has always been a leading cause of death. The 2023 global tuberculosis report by WHO showed 7.5 million new TB cases diagnosed and an estimated 1.3 million deaths (about 17.3% mortality) in 2022, leading to a tremendous social and economic burden. Multidrug-resistant TB (MDR-TB) is TB that is resistant to rifampicin and isoniazid and was supposed to be the main block of global TB control. Then, the incidence data of MDR-TB and rifampicin-resistant tuberculosis (RR-TB) in China is the fourth in the world. The treatment process of MDR-TB is very long and expensive, leading to a decrease in individual patients' compliance and an increase in economic burden [1]. At the same time, the occurrence of MDR-TB aggravated the control of MTB, making the treatment situation dire [2]. Although the clinical diagnostic rate of MTB has improved, some TB patients can be misdiagnosed. The occurrence of MDR-TB was primarily associated with inaccurate clinical diagnosis, overuse of antibiotics, patient non-compliance, and intrinsic drug resistance mutations of MTB. Therefore, rapid identification of tuberculosis infection and drug resistance types is crucial to curb the current high incidence rate, high mortality, and high economic burden of tuberculosis. Although many studies have stated the risk factors of MDR-TB, with inconsistent or conflicting results, the medication history was considered the leading risk factor of MDR-TB. As a developing country, China has a vast territory and relatively unbalanced economic development. There are significant differences in tuberculosis prevalence, distribution, risk factors, and characteristics of MDR-TB in different regions. The understanding of the status quo and prevalence, mechanisms, and countermeasures of antibiotic resistance of MTB is of great significance for controlling *Mycobacterium tuberculosis*, which plays a beneficial role in guiding the formulation of national and local public health policies.

2. The prevalence of MTB

2.1 High incidence and prevalence

As one of the major infectious diseases in the world, the incidence and prevalence of tuberculosis have been a concern for the public health sector. In 2022, there were an estimated 10.6 million TB people worldwide. From 2020 to 2022, the TB incidence rate sustained growth in the region of Southeast Asia, the Americas, and the Western Pacific. The former three regions that developed TB were Southeast Asia (46%), Africa (23%), and the Western Pacific (18%). India (27%), Indonesia (10%), China (7.1%), the Philippines (7.0%), and Pakistan (5.7%) were the top five of 30 high TB burden countries, which accounted for more than half of all estimated incident cases worldwide [3]. From the Global Tuberculosis Report 2023, there were 12.4 thousand confirmed cases of multidrug-resistant/rifampin-resistant tuberculosis (MDR-TB/RR-TB) in China, and the treatment success rate was only 51%.

Across the MTB data from 2005 to 2016 in mainland China [4], the mean incidence of pulmonary TB (PTB) was 66.61 per 100,000 population and the former three high mean annual incidences of MTB was Xinjiang Uygur Autonomous Region (135.03 per 100,000 population), Guizhou Province (115.98 per 100,000 population), and the Tibet Autonomous Region (101.98 per 100,000 population). Other data also showed that the incidence of MTB in the western region (such as counties in Xinjiang, Guizhou, and Tibet) was significantly higher than that in the eastern and central areas of mainland China [5]. These high incidence regions also had relatively low declining trends compared to the other areas. The relatively low economic level and scarcity of resources for medical service systems and facilities were associated with the high incidence of PTB in the western region of China, due to the inability to receive a diagnosis and treatment in a timely manner.

2.2 Population distribution

Males had a higher prevalence rate than females, and the 75–79 years age group showed the highest prevalence [3]. This finding was consistent with the Global TB Reports 2022 and 2023. Jiang et al. reported that MTB patients were predominantly male (69.8%) and farmers or herders (70.0%), with a total of 10,582,903 patients [4]. Those 60 years or older were the highest population, with MTB accounting for 28.53%. Zhou et al. [6] showed that the majority of patients with resistant pulmonary tuberculosis were farmers, probably influenced by cultural and environmental factors, and students were more likely to be infected with MTB. The male and elderly male may be more likely to suffer MTB in China, probably due to tobacco use, corticosteroid use, immunity levels, migration, and living environment [4]. Reinforcement of the related control education and screen frequency for TB should be taken to decrease this preference among males.

2.3 Prevalence regions

The prevalence of MDR-TB has prominent regional characteristics, mainly in the following regions: India, China, and Pakistan [3]. A study by Yu et al. showed that the TB prevalence was distributed primarily in the southeast of Chongqing, which covered three counties and two districts (Xiushan County, Youyang County, Pengshui County, Qianjiang District, and Wulong District). The annual average notification rate and pathogenic positive of pulmonary tuberculosis were 79/100,000 population and 25/100,000 population in Chongqing, China, 2011–2018, respectively [7]. Another study in Chongqing from 2016 to 2022 was reported, showing a total of 9920 student TB cases with an average incidence rate of 24.89/100,000. High school students (age: 13–18 years; 6649/9920, 67.03%) and college students accounted for the majority of PTB cases, and prevalence regions were predominantly located in the southeast and northeast parts of Chongqing, consistent with the study [7, 8]. The research by Lv et al. showed that males exhibited higher disability-adjusted life years than females with MDR-TB [3]. The possible cause of the higher incidence among males may be due to their more extensive activity range and more frequent interactions with peers [8]. Yin et al. [9] analyzed the recent transmission of MTB in Lianyungang, Jiangsu province of China, over 10 years. The result showed spatial aggregation of TB transmission located in Haizhou, Donghai, and Guanyun. Another study in Shanghai showed that geographical aggregation of MTB could be linked to genotypic clustering [10].

The above research showed the prevalence situation of different regions, mainly associated with the backwards economy, shortage of health resources, and local government interventions, leading to an inability to afford the diagnosis and treatment of TB. Then, the reason for the higher PTB risks of high school and college students compared to younger students could be attributed to the limitation of Bacillus Calmette-Guérin vaccine protection over time [11]. At the same time, there are some common characteristics in different regions, and also regional characteristics, which also confirms the necessity of TB epidemiological characteristics investigation and regional public health policy formulation.

2.4 Infectiousness of pulmonary TB

The infectivity of tuberculosis is an effective means to evaluate the treatment plan and treatment effect on patients, and it is related to many factors. The newest studies suggested that the infectiousness of people with pulmonary TB was associated with the sputum smear positivity, culture time-to-positivity, Xpert MTB/RIF cycle threshold value, detection of MTB from cough aerosol, and face mask sampling. Clinical factors, such as cough strength, frequency and cavitation, affect infectiousness, and effective treatment rapidly decreases infectiousness [12]. Another study showed that 83.81% (233/278) of MDR/RR-TB cases were likely caused by transmission from 2019 to 2021 data in Sichuan, China. MTB with the KatG S315T amino acid substitution presented a higher risk of transmission of MDR/RR-TB [13]. The clustering risk decreased with increasing distances of TB patients [14].

2.5 Risk factors for MTB

As is known to all, TB tends to occur in people with weakened immune systems, such as those with immune system diseases, HIV, diabetes mellitus (DM), cancer, the elderly, and immunosuppressant users [15]. In addition, people with close contact with TB, chronic lung disease, poor nutrition and hygiene, smoking and alcohol abuse, and depression are also generally susceptible. HIV-1 infection is the most significant risk factor for MTB infection. HIV could increase the possibility of endogenous recurrence and exogenous reinfection of MTB. In addition, MTB increases the occurrence of HIV-1 replication and chronic immune activation, accelerating the progression of HIV-1 disease [16]. Xiaoxiao Cai et al. [17] research showed the risk factor of drug-resistant tuberculosis patients with and without diabetes mellitus difference: residence in rural areas, retreatment of tuberculosis, pulmonary cavity, and uric acid ≥346 μmol/L identified as independent risk factors for MDR-TB without DM, and residence in rural areas, retreatment of tuberculosis, pulmonary cavity, and HbA1c ≥ 9.8% as independent risk factors for MDR-TB with DM.

At the same time, tuberculosis is a chronic wasting disease, and the disease itself can also damage the body's immunity, leading to more serious disease progression. Therefore, improving immunity and avoiding bad living habits can not only reduce the risk of contracting TB but also enhance the effectiveness of treatment for TB patients. Recently, a retrospective multicenter cohort study in China showed that smoking history, baseline sputum acid-fast bacilli smear-positive, lung cavities, bilateral disease, previous anti-tuberculosis treatment, or comorbidity of viral hepatitis could impact the faster culture conversion in MDR-TB patients. In contrast, the anti-tuberculosis drug of bedaquiline was contrary [18]. A study from Shanghai [10] showed local transmission between both migrants and residents induced the urban center incidence of TB. A TB study in Hunan province demonstrated that males, aged 30–60 years, ethnic minorities, nonfarmers, retreated TB patients, and MDR/RR-TB were independent risk factors for TB transmission [19]. The evaluation of risk factors for MTB was helpful to formulate a pertinent policy and make clear the direction of the tuberculosis strategy.

3. Drug resistance profile of MTB

Anti-tuberculosis drugs are divided into first-line and second-line drugs. First-line anti-tuberculosis drugs include isoniazid, rifampicin, ethambutol, streptomycin, and pyrazinamide. In contrast, second-line anti-tuberculosis drugs include levofloxacin, moxifloxacin, bedaquinoline, linezolid, cycloserine, capreomycin, clofazimine, delamanid, amikacin, aminosalicylic acid, etc. Anti-TB first-line medicines are mainly used for the treatment of non-drug-resistant TB, and second-line anti-TB drugs are used primarily for the treatment of drug-resistant TB. The WHO Global TB Report 2023 divides TB into five categories based on the resistance of *Mycobacterium tuberculosis* to antibiotics: Isonazid-resistant tuberculosis (IR-TB), RR-TB, MDR-TB, Pre-XDR-TB, and XDR-TB. MDR-TB is defined as resistance to rifampicin and isoniazid. Pre-XDR-TB is TB that is resistant to rifampicin and any fluoroquinolone (a class of second-line anti-TB drugs). XDR-TB is TB that is resistant to rifampicin, plus any fluoroquinolone, plus at least one of either bedaquiline or linezolid. Detection of resistance to isoniazid and rifampicin is a key basis for judging drug-resistant/multidrug-resistant TB.

Drugs	**Drug resistance genes**	**Resistance rate (%)**
First-line anti-tuberculosis drugs		
Rifampicin	*rpoA, rpoB, rpoC, rpoZ, Rv2752c* [21–24], *ponA1* [25]	8.6–38.7 [24, 26–28]
Isoniazid	*katG, fabG1, inhA, ahpC, ndh, kasA, Rv1258c, Rv2752c* [22–24, 29]	16.4–49.0 [24, 26, 27]
Streptomycin	*rrs, rpsL, gidB* [30]	4.2–31.0 [31, 32]
Ethambutol	*embA, embB, embC, embR, ropC, ubiA, aftA* [33–35],	4.1–20.7 [26, 31, 32]
Pyrazinamide	*rpsA, PncA, panD* [36]	3.4–11.6 [31]
Second-line anti-tuberculosis drugs		
Levofloxacin/LEV	*gyrA, gyrB* [23]	12.9–17.6 [27, 37]
Moxifloxacin/MXF	*gyrA, gyrB* [23]	13.2–13.7 [27, 37]
Bedaquiline	*Rv0678, atpE, pepQ, Rv2535c, rv1979c, mmpL5, mmpS5, Rv3249c* [23, 38–41]	0.4–0.9 [27, 42]
linezolid	*rrl, rplC, Rv3249c* [23, 43–45]	1.3–3.1 [27, 46]
Cycloserine	*Ald, Alr, ddlA*, ald [47, 48]	1.8–29.8 [49, 50]
Capreomycin	*tlya, rrs, eis, gidB* [51–53]	1.7 [50]
Clofazimine	*Rv0678, Rv1979c, Rv2535c, pepQ* [54, 55]	15.4 [49]
Delamanid	*Ddn, fbiA, fbiB, fbiC, fgd1* [56–60]	2.1 [49]
Amikacin	rrs, whiB7, gid, eis [61]	2.2 [50]
Aminosalicylic acid	dfrA, folC, ribD, thyA, thyX [62–64]	4.6 [50]
Ethionamide	*ethA, ethR, inhA* [65]	11.3 [50]

Table 1.
List of resistance rates of anti-tuberculosis drugs.

The drug resistance mechanism of MTB is divided into intrinsic and acquired resistance. Inherent drug resistance mainly includes three points: reduced cell wall permeability, changed efflux pump function, and affected cell metabolism. The primary drug resistance mechanism to MTB is the mutations in target genes. Moreover, the poor treatment compliance of TB patients, treatment interruption, co-infection with other diseases (diabetes, HIV, liver diseases, immune system diseases, etc.), large-scale population movement, and other factors have aggravated the emergence and spread of drug-resistant strains of TB, resulting in treatment failure of TB patients, and increasing the burden of treatment in low- and middle-income countries [20]. To better understand the drug resistance of tuberculosis, the researchers summarized the drug resistance genes and drug resistance rates of some anti-tuberculosis drugs by referring to the literature and data to treat tuberculosis better (**Table 1**).

From **Table 1**, we can see that the drug resistance genes and resistance rates varied and that resistance surveillance was necessary. As a whole, the line one anti-tuberculosis drug resistance rates are relatively higher than the line two anti-tuberculosis drug resistance rates. Then, the treatment of tuberculosis faces pain points, such as long cycles, high drug resistance rate, and prolonged drug sensitivity reporting time, which brings great trouble to the diagnosis and treatment of tuberculosis. The diversity of diagnostic methods provides more selectivity for diagnosing and treating tuberculosis, but the sensitivity and specificity still need to be improved. Therefore, the road to ending tuberculosis is obstacle-packed and long.

4. Control and prevention of MDR-TB infections

Early diagnosis is an essential means to detect drug-resistant tuberculosis. Surveillance of key populations (e.g., people with TB/HIV co-infection, the elderly, people with diabetes, people having close contact with TB patients, mobile populations) and in key settings (e.g., nursing homes/homes for the aged, schools, psychiatric hospitals) is an essential means of stopping the occurrence and spread of TB outbreaks. At the same time, improving the diagnostic efficiency of drug-resistant TB is also critical for the early diagnosis of TB. With low sensitivity and long turnaround time, the conventional smear microscopy technique and bacterial culture method cannot satisfy the accurate diagnosis of MDR-TB. WHO recommends GeneXpert MTB/RIF Ultra as an essential test for drug-resistant TB, but it cannot achieve full coverage of all drug-resistant TB types. Because of the high cost of the equipment, GeneXpert MTB/RIF Ultra was only used in certified hospitals in urban areas, and it is rarely used in rural areas. The next-generation sequencing approach has been a valuable diagnostic tool for detecting MTB, with a sensitivity of 94.64% and specificity of 98.94% [66]. Although next-generation sequencing is a valuable tool to predict MTB drug resistance, the limitations of long turnaround time and high cost make it unfriendly to the diagnosis of MTB [67]. It is worth our attention that many researchers have made use of emerging technologies, such as matrix-assisted laser desorption/ionization time-of-flight technology, clustered regularly interspaced short palindromic repeats technology, droplet digital PCR technology, microfluidic technology, gene chip technology, etc., to achieve the diagnosis of drug-resistant TB, which has a vital role in promoting the diagnosis of drug-resistant TB.

Standardized diagnosis and treatment are an essential guarantee to control and prevent the spread of drug-resistant TB. To eliminate the bacterium, TB is treatable with combined antibiotics, usually lasting 6 to 9 months or more. Thus, developing novel anti-tubercular drugs with various structural classes is necessary to solve the problems [68]. The development of new anti-tuberculosis drugs often focuses on MTB cell wall synthesis and the identification of drug targets. Shahin et al. showed that decaprenylphosphoryl-β-D-ribose-2-epimerase (DprE) inhibitors reduce DPA formation, leading to MTB cell death [69]. Gao et al. suggested a model for Rv3806c-catalyzed phosphoribose transfer through an inverting mechanism, with potential for new anti-tuberculosis drug development [70]. Kassem et al. revealed that a series of coumarins could inhibit the InhA enzyme and MTB cell growth [71]. The treatment of tuberculosis follows the principle of "early, combined, appropriate, regular and whole course". Different types of TB treatment plans vary and should be carried out in strict accordance with the recommended drug regimen and guidelines. At the same time, sputum smear, peripheral blood cells, urine routine, liver function, kidney function, blood glucose, chest imaging, electrocardiogram, vision examination, and drug-resistant tuberculosis should be monitored during treatment. Strengthening health education is an important measure to improve the cure rate of drug-resistant tuberculosis and prevent the spread of tuberculosis bacilli. Strengthening health education for TB patients and family members, improving bad behavior habits, strengthening nutrition, and forming a good lifestyle are vital to improving the cure rate of drug-resistant TB and preventing the spread of drug-resistant TB. Research on the prevalence, risk factors, and drug resistance profiles of MTB is of great significance for the formulation of treatment plans for TB patients and the evaluation of treatment effects, and it will promote the global strategy of curbing the spread of drug-resistant TB and finally ending TB in future.

Funding statement

This work was funded by the Fifth People's Hospital of Huai'an Collaboration Foundation (Grant No. HWY-YL-20230072).

Conflict of interest

The authors declare that the research was conducted without any commercial or financial relationships that could be construed as a potential conflict of interest.

Author details

Xue-Song Xiong[1†], Qin-Hui Zhu[1†], Zhan-Zhong Liu[2], Ting-Ting Huang[1], Jin-Bin Fan[3], Xiao Zhao[1], Jian-Song Gu[1*] and Fen Li[1*]

1 The Fifth People's Hospital of Huai'an (Huai'an Hospital Affiliate to Yangzhou University), Huai'an, Jiangsu Province, China

2 Xuzhou Infectious Diseases Hospital, Xuzhou, Jiangsu Province, China

3 Department of Laboratory Medicine, Suqian Hospital of Traditional Chinese Medicine, Suqian, Jiangsu Province, China

*Address all correspondence to: 876448066@qq.com and 3063892835@qq.com

† These authors contributed equally to the study.

References

[1] Wang DM, Liu H, Zheng YL, Xu YH, Liao Y. Epidemiology of nontuberculous *Mycobacteria* in tuberculosis suspects, southwest of China, 2017-2022. Frontiers in Cellular and Infection Microbiology. 2023;**13**:1282902

[2] Yu JJ, Tang SJ. Annual progress of chemotherapy of multidrug/rifampicin-resistant tuberculosis in 2022. Zhonghua Jie He He Hu Xi Za Zhi. 2023;**46**(1):62-66

[3] Lv H, Zhang X, Zhang X, et al. Global prevalence and burden of multidrug-resistant tuberculosis from 1990 to 2019. BMC Infectious Diseases. 2024;**24**(1):243

[4] Jiang H, Liu M, Zhang Y, et al. Changes in incidence and epidemiological characteristics of pulmonary tuberculosis in mainland China, 2005-2016. JAMA Network Open. 2021;**4**(4):e215302

[5] Hu M, Feng Y, Li T, et al. Unbalanced risk of pulmonary tuberculosis in China at the subnational scale: Spatiotemporal analysis. JMIR Public Health and Surveillance. 2022;**8**(7):e36242

[6] Zhou J, Li J, Hu Y, Li S. Epidemiological characteristics, diagnosis and treatment effect of rifampicin-resistant pulmonary tuberculosis (RR-PTB) in Guizhou Province. BMC Infectious Diseases. 2024;**24**(1):1058

[7] Yu Y, Wu B, Wu C, Wang Q, Hu D, Chen W. Spatial-temporal analysis of tuberculosis in Chongqing, China 2011-2018. BMC Infectious Diseases. 2020;**20**(1):531

[8] Kong D, Wu C, Cui Y, et al. Epidemiological characteristics and spatiotemporal clustering of pulmonary tuberculosis among students in Southwest China from 2016 to 2022: Analysis of population-based surveillance data. JMIR Public Health and Surveillance. 2024;**10**:e64286

[9] Yin X, Zhang Q, Wang Y, et al. Genomic and spatial analysis on the recent transmission of *Mycobacterium tuberculosis* in Eastern China: A 10-year retrospective population-based study. Infection and Drug Resistance. 2024;**17**:4257-4269

[10] Yang C, Lu L, Warren JL, et al. Internal migration and transmission dynamics of tuberculosis in Shanghai, China: An epidemiological, spatial, genomic analysis. The Lancet Infectious Diseases. 2018;**18**(7):788-795

[11] Huang W, Fang Z, Luo S, et al. The effect of BCG vaccination and risk factors for latent tuberculosis infection among college freshmen in China. International Journal of Infectious Diseases. 2022;**122**:321-6.2

[12] Nathavitharana RR, Pearl A, Biewer A, et al. Assessing infectiousness and the impact of effective treatment to guide isolation recommendations for people with pulmonary tuberculosis. The Journal of Infectious Diseases. 2025;**231**(1):10-22

[13] Gao W, Wang W, Li J, et al. Drug-resistance characteristics, genetic diversity, and transmission dynamics of multidrug-resistant or rifampicin-resistant *Mycobacterium tuberculosis* from 2019 to 2021 in Sichuan, China. Antimicrobial Resistance and Infection Control. 2024;**13**(1):125

[14] Quan Z, Xu J, Li M, et al. Transmission of tuberculosis in rural

Henan, China: A prospective population-based genomic spatial epidemiological study. Emerging Microbes & Infections. 2024;**13**(1):2399273

[15] Jarde A, Romano E, Afaq S, et al. Prevalence and risks of tuberculosis multimorbidity in low-income and middle-income countries: A meta-review. BMJ Open. 2022;**12**(9):e060906

[16] Han X, Wang X, Han F, et al. The cGAS-STING pathway in HIV-1 and *Mycobacterium tuberculosis* coinfection. Infection. 2025;**53**(2):495-511

[17] Cai X, Xu X, He G, Jiang X, Wu L. Drug resistance in drug-resistant tuberculosis patients with and without diabetes mellitus: A comparative analysis. BMC Infectious Diseases. 2024;**24**(1):807

[18] Chen Q, He W, Du J, et al. Predictors of early and interim culture un-conversion in multidrug-resistant/rifampicin-resistant tuberculosis: A retrospective multi-center cohort study in China. Antimicrobial Resistance and Infection Control. 2024;**13**(1):126

[19] He W, Tan Y, Song Z, et al. Transmission dynamics of tuberculosis in a high-burden area of China: An 8-year population-based study using whole genome sequencing. International Journal of Infectious Diseases. 2024;**147**:107210

[20] Zhiteng Y, Fei R, Hua W, et al. Analysis of influencing factors of treatment outcomes of retreated multidrug resistant/rifampicin-resistant pulmonary tuberculosis patients: A national multicenter retrospective cohort study. Chinese Journal of Antituberculosis; 1-14

[21] Nusrath Unissa A, Hassan S, Indira Kumari V, Revathy R, Hanna LE. Insights into RpoB clinical mutants in mediating rifampicin resistance in *Mycobacterium tuberculosis*. Journal of Molecular Graphics & Modelling. 2016;**67**:20-32

[22] Garcia-Marin AM, Cancino-Munoz I, Torres-Puente M, et al. Role of the first WHO mutation catalogue in the diagnosis of antibiotic resistance in *Mycobacterium tuberculosis* in the Valencia region, Spain: A retrospective genomic analysis. Lancet Microbe. 2024;**5**(1):e43-e51

[23] Consortium CR. Quantitative measurement of antibiotic resistance in *Mycobacterium tuberculosis* reveals genetic determinants of resistance and susceptibility in a target gene approach. Nature Communications. 2024;**15**(1):488

[24] Napier G, Campino S, Phelan JE, Clark TG. Large-scale genomic analysis of *Mycobacterium tuberculosis* reveals extent of target and compensatory mutations linked to multi-drug resistant tuberculosis. Scientific Reports. 2023;**13**(1):623

[25] Qadir M, Khan MT, Khan SA, et al. Unveiling the complexity of rifampicin drug susceptibility testing in *Mycobacterium tuberculosis*: Comparative analysis with next-generation sequencing. Journal of Medical Microbiology. 2024;**73**(9)

[26] Jin C, Wu Y, Chen J, et al. Prevalence and patterns of drug-resistant *Mycobacterium tuberculosis* in newly diagnosed patients in China: A systematic review and meta-analysis. Journal of Global Antimicrobial Resistance. 2024;**38**:292-301

[27] The CC. A data compendium associating the genomes of 12,289 *Mycobacterium tuberculosis* isolates with quantitative resistance phenotypes to 13 antibiotics. PLoS Biology. 2022;**20**(8):e3001721

[28] Yan Y, Xiangrong Z. Correlation between isoniazid-resistant gene mutation and drug resistance level in Mycobacterium tuberculosis. Journal of Nanjing Medical University (Natural Sciences). 2023;**43**(03):392-396

[29] Seifert M, Catanzaro D, Catanzaro A, Rodwell TC. Genetic mutations associated with isoniazid resistance in *Mycobacterium tuberculosis*: A systematic review. PLoS One. 2015;**10**(3):e0119628

[30] Bifani P, Mathema B, Campo M, et al. Molecular identification of streptomycin monoresistant *Mycobacterium tuberculosis* related to multidrug-resistant W strain. Emerging Infectious Diseases. 2001;**7**(5):842-848

[31] Thomsen J, Abdulrazzaq NM, Nyasulu PS, et al. Epidemiology and antimicrobial resistance of *Mycobacterium* spp. in the United Arab Emirates: A retrospective analysis of 12 years of national antimicrobial resistance surveillance data. Frontiers in Public Health. 2024;**12**:1244353

[32] Soliman MS, Hansen CH, Hanafy M, et al. Drug resistance and genomic variations among *Mycobacterium tuberculosis* isolates from The Nile Delta, Egypt. Scientific Reports. 2024;**14**(1):20401

[33] Ramaswamy SV, Amin AG, Göksel S, et al. Molecular genetic analysis of nucleotide polymorphisms associated with ethambutol resistance in human isolates of *Mycobacterium tuberculosis*. Antimicrobial Agents and Chemotherapy. 2000;**44**(2):326-336

[34] Brossier F, Sougakoff W, Bernard C, et al. Molecular analysis of the embCAB locus and embR gene involved in ethambutol resistance in clinical isolates of *Mycobacterium tuberculosis* in France. Antimicrobial Agents and Chemotherapy. 2015;**59**(8):4800-4808

[35] Xu Y, Jia H, Huang H, Sun Z, Zhang Z. Mutations found in embCAB, embR, and ubiA genes of ethambutol-sensitive and -resistant *Mycobacterium tuberculosis* clinical isolates from China. BioMed Research International. 2015;**2015**:951706

[36] Werngren J, Alm E, Mansjö M. Non-pncA gene-mutated but pyrazinamide-resistant *Mycobacterium tuberculosis*: Why is that? Journal of Clinical Microbiology. 2017;**55**(6):1920-1927

[37] Li S, Tan Y, Deng Y, et al. The emerging threat of fluroquinolone-, bedaquiline-, and linezolid-resistant *Mycobacterium tuberculosis* in China: Observations on surveillance data. Journal of Infection and Public Health. 2024;**17**(1):137-142

[38] Nguyen TVA, Anthony RM, Bañuls AL, Nguyen TVA, Vu DH, Alffenaar JC. Bedaquiline resistance: Its emergence, mechanism, and prevention. Clinical Infectious Diseases. 2018;**66**(10):1625-1630

[39] Saeed DK, Shakoor S, Razzak SA, et al. Variants associated with Bedaquiline (BDQ) resistance identified in Rv0678 and efflux pump genes in *Mycobacterium tuberculosis* isolates from BDQ naïve TB patients in Pakistan. BMC Microbiology. 2022;**22**(1):62

[40] Beckert P, Sanchez-Padilla E, Merker M, et al. MDR *M. Tuberculosis* outbreak clone in Eswatini missed by Xpert has elevated bedaquiline resistance dated to the pre-treatment era. Genome Medicine. 2020;**12**(1):104

[41] Derendinger B, Dippenaar A, de Vos M, et al. Bedaquiline resistance in

patients with drug-resistant tuberculosis in Cape Town, South Africa: A retrospective longitudinal cohort study. Lancet Microbe. 2023;**4**(12):e972-ee82

[42] He W, Liu C, Liu D, et al. Prevalence of *Mycobacterium tuberculosis* resistant to bedaquiline and delamanid in China. Journal of Global Antimicrobial Resistance. 2021;**26**:241-248

[43] Hillemann D, Rüsch-Gerdes S, Richter E. In vitro-selected linezolid-resistant *Mycobacterium tuberculosis* mutants. Antimicrobial Agents and Chemotherapy. 2008;**52**(2):800-801

[44] Zimenkov DV, Nosova EY, Kulagina EV, et al. Examination of bedaquiline- and linezolid-resistant *Mycobacterium tuberculosis* isolates from the Moscow region. The Journal of Antimicrobial Chemotherapy. 2017;**72**(7):1901-1906

[45] Zong Z, Jing W, Shi J, et al. Comparison of in vitro activity and MIC distributions between the novel oxazolidinone delpazolid and linezolid against multidrug-resistant and extensively drug-resistant *Mycobacterium tuberculosis* in China. Antimicrobial Agents and Chemotherapy. 2018;**62**(8):e00165-18

[46] Nambiar R, Tornheim JA, Diricks M, et al. Linezolid resistance in *Mycobacterium tuberculosis* isolates at a tertiary care Centre in Mumbai, India. The Indian Journal of Medical Research. 2021;**154**(1):85-89

[47] Desjardins CA, Cohen KA, Munsamy V, et al. Genomic and functional analyses of *Mycobacterium tuberculosis* strains implicate ald in D-cycloserine resistance. Nature Genetics. 2016;**48**(5):544-551

[48] Belanger AE, Porter JC, Hatfull GF. Genetic analysis of peptidoglycan biosynthesis in mycobacteria: Characterization of a ddlA mutant of *Mycobacterium smegmatis*. Journal of Bacteriology. 2000;**182**(23):6854-6856

[49] Trisakul K, Nonghanphithak D, Chaiyachat P, et al. High clustering rate and genotypic drug-susceptibility screening for the newly recommended anti-tuberculosis drugs among global extensively drug-resistant *Mycobacterium tuberculosis* isolates. Emerging Microbes & Infections. 2022;**11**(1):1857-1866

[50] Khademi F, Sahebkar A. An updated systematic review and meta-analysis on *Mycobacterium tuberculosis* antibiotic resistance in Iran (2013-2020). Iranian Journal of Basic Medical Sciences. 2021;**24**(4):428-436

[51] Maus CE, Plikaytis BB, Shinnick TM. Molecular analysis of cross-resistance to capreomycin, kanamycin, amikacin, and viomycin in *Mycobacterium tuberculosis*. Antimicrobial Agents and Chemotherapy. 2005;**49**(8):3192-3197

[52] Maus CE, Plikaytis BB, Shinnick TM. Mutation of tlyA confers capreomycin resistance in *Mycobacterium tuberculosis*. Antimicrobial Agents and Chemotherapy. 2005;**49**(2):571-577

[53] Jugheli L, Bzekalava N, de Rijk P, Fissette K, Portaels F, Rigouts L. High level of cross-resistance between kanamycin, amikacin, and capreomycin among *Mycobacterium tuberculosis* isolates from Georgia and a close relation with mutations in the rrs gene. Antimicrobial Agents and Chemotherapy. 2009;**53**(12):5064-5068

[54] Xu J, Wang B, Hu M, et al. Primary clofazimine and bedaquiline resistance among isolates from patients with multidrug-resistant tuberculosis. Antimicrobial Agents and Chemotherapy. 2017;**61**(6):e00239-17

[55] Chauhan A, Kumar M, Kumar A, Kanchan K. Comprehensive review on mechanism of action, resistance and evolution of antimycobacterial drugs. Life Sciences. 2021;**274**:119301

[56] Nguyen QT, Trinco G, Binda C, Mattevi A, Fraaije MW. Discovery and characterization of an F(420)-dependent glucose-6-phosphate dehydrogenase (Rh-FGD1) from *Rhodococcus jostii* RHA1. Applied Microbiology and Biotechnology. 2017;**101**(7):2831-2842

[57] Xavier AS, Lakshmanan M. Delamanid: A new armor in combating drug-resistant tuberculosis. Journal of Pharmacology and Pharmacotherapeutics. 2014;**5**(3):222-224

[58] Manjunatha UH, Boshoff H, Dowd CS, et al. Identification of a nitroimidazo-oxazine-specific protein involved in PA-824 resistance in *Mycobacterium tuberculosis*. Proceedings of the National Academy of Sciences of the United States of America. 2006;**103**(2):431-436

[59] Forouhar F, Abashidze M, Xu H, et al. Molecular insights into the biosynthesis of the F420 coenzyme. The Journal of Biological Chemistry. 2008;**283**(17):11832-11840

[60] Bashiri G, Rehan AM, Sreebhavan S, Baker HM, Baker EN, Squire CJ. Elongation of the poly-γ-glutamate tail of F420 requires both domains of the F420: Γ-Glutamyl ligase (FbiB) of *Mycobacterium tuberculosis*. The Journal of Biological Chemistry. 2016;**291**(13):6882-6894

[61] Finci I, Albertini A, Merker M, et al. Investigating resistance in clinical *Mycobacterium tuberculosis* complex isolates with genomic and phenotypic antimicrobial susceptibility testing: A multicentre observational study. Lancet Microbe. 2022;**3**(9):e672-ee82

[62] Zhang Y, Wang S, Chen X, Cui P, Chen J, Zhang W. Mutations in the promoter region of methionine transporter gene metM (Rv3253c) confer Para-aminosalicylic acid (PAS) resistance in *Mycobacterium tuberculosis*. MBio. 2024;**15**(2):e0207323

[63] Wang W, Li S, Ge Q, et al. Determination of critical concentration for drug susceptibility testing of *Mycobacterium tuberculosis* against Para-aminosalicylic acid with clinical isolates with thyA, folC and dfrA mutations. Annals of Clinical Microbiology and Antimicrobials. 2022;**21**(1):48

[64] Dokladda K, Billamas P, Jaitrong S, et al. Whole genome sequencing reveals candidate genes involving in PAS resistance in *M. Tuberculosis* isolated from patients in Thailand. World Journal of Microbiology and Biotechnology. 2023;**40**(1):32

[65] Maitre T, Morel F, Brossier F, et al. How a PCR sequencing strategy can bring new data to improve the diagnosis of ethionamide resistance. Microorganisms. 2022;**10**(7):1436

[66] Xiao H, Zhou C, Xiao Z, et al. Metagenomic next-generation sequencing of bronchoalveolar lavage fluid samples offers diagnostic utility in bacteriologically negative pulmonary tuberculosis. Diagnostic Microbiology and Infectious Disease. 2025;**111**(4):116725

[67] Xiong XS, Zhang XD, Yan JW, et al. Identification of *Mycobacterium tuberculosis* resistance to common antibiotics: An overview of current methods and techniques. Infection and Drug Resistance. 2024;**17**:1491-1506

[68] Sahoo BM, Nandi P, Sahu DR, et al. Microwave-assisted green synthesis: An approach for the development of

anti-tubercular agents. Current Drug Targets; 2025

[69] Fil M, Alibert S. Unveiling DprE1 as a key target in the fight against tuberculosis: Insights and perspectives on developing novel antimicrobial agents. BioMed. 2024;**4**(3):220-236

[70] Gao S, Wu F, Gurcha SS, et al. Structural analysis of phosphoribosyltransferase-mediated cell wall precursor synthesis in *Mycobacterium tuberculosis*. Nature Microbiology. 2024;**9**(4):976-987

[71] Kassem AF, Sabt A, Korycka-Machala M, et al. New coumarin linked thiazole derivatives as antimycobacterial agents: Design, synthesis, enoyl acyl carrier protein reductase (InhA) inhibition and molecular modeling. Bioorganic Chemistry. 2024;**150**:107511

Section 2

Antibiotic Resistance and Pathogenesis

Chapter 3

Antibiotic Resistance in Mycobacteria

Jumei Zeng, Xingyan Tan and Chao Gao

Abstract

Mycobacterium infection caused by *Mycobacterium tuberculosis* (MTB) and non-tuberculosis mycobacterium (NTM) presents a serious threat to global health, mainly due to a protracted treatment regimen involving a combination of drugs. Antibiotic resistance in mycobacterium is mainly due to a frequent gene mutation that encodes antibiotic resistance. There are also several additional unique features of drug resistance, such as chromosomal mutation, efflux pumps, bacterial heterogeneity, slow metabolism, biofilm formation, antibiotic degradation or modification, target modification, and host microenvironment. In this chapter, we discuss the traditional mechanisms of drug resistance in mycobacterium, newer understandings, and the shaping of unconventional approaches to target both the emergence and treatment of drug resistance in mycobacterium.

Keywords: *Mycobacterium tuberculosis*, non-tuberculous mycobacteria (NTM), anti-TB drug, antibiotic, gene mutation, efflux pump, cell wall envelope, resistance, tolerance

1. Introduction

Currently, worldwide efforts in mycobacterial infection control encounter significant challenges due to antibiotic resistance. The extensive clinical use of antituberculosis drugs has facilitated the global proliferation of multidrug-resistant tuberculosis (MDR-TB) and extensively drug-resistant tuberculosis (XDR-TB), complicating the tuberculosis control measures due to the challenges posed by antimicrobial resistance. According to *the WHO Global Tuberculosis Report 2023*, approximately 410,000 individuals were reported to have drug-resistant tuberculosis in 2022, resulting in around 160,000 fatalities [1]. Infections caused by non-tuberculosis mycobacterium (NTM) are generally not mandated to be reported [2], leading to a deficiency of comprehensive data on resistance patterns. Nonetheless, such infections are notorious for their diagnostic challenges, difficulties in treatment, and innate resistance to various antibiotics. This chapter will elucidate the innate and acquired mechanisms of antibiotic resistance in mycobacteria, as shown in **Figure 1**, as well as explore strategies to transcend this challenge and the development of novel approaches, both of which are crucial for effective therapeutic intervention.

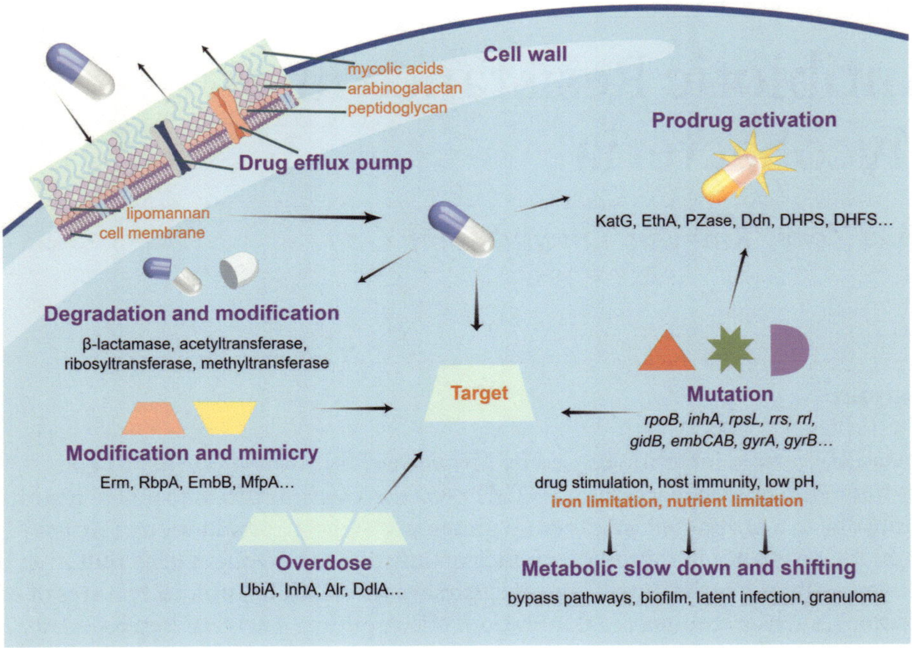

Figure 1.
Drug resistance mechanisms in mycobacterium. Note. Key processes include the structural components of the cell wall, the role of drug efflux pumps, and various enzymatic modifications that degrade or mimic drug action. Additionally, we highlight the significance of prodrug activation, mutations in target genes, and metabolic adaptations that contribute to resistance.

2. Innate resistance mechanism

Mycobacteria exhibit intrinsic resistance to various commonly used antibiotics, posing a significant challenge in clinical treatment. This inherent resistance is attributable to mycobacteria's unique structural and genetic characteristics. The high lipid contents of their cell wall contribute to their impermeability to drugs. Additionally, the genome encodes a range of inherent resistance determinants, including β-lactamases, acetyltransferases, other enzymes responsible for drug degradation and modification, and efflux systems [3–6]. A comprehensive understanding of these resistance mechanisms will facilitate the appropriate implementation of existing therapeutic strategies and advance the conceptualization of novel treatment approaches.

2.1 Peculiar characteristics of the mycobacterial cell wall

Mycobacteria possess a highly complex and unique cell envelope, which consists of a peptidoglycan layer, a mycolic acid layer, and an arabinogalactan polysaccharide. This envelope protects and assists the growth of the bacteria and allows their adaptation to the host. Phylogenetically, mycobacteria are closely related to gram-positive bacteria and possess many typical characteristics of this group [7]. The mycolic acid-peptidoglycan-arabinogalactan complex is the core of the cell wall, with various lipopolysaccharides and lipids, such as lipoarabinomannan, trehalose dimycolate, and phenolic glycolipids non-covalently anchored to the core [8]. Like conventional gram-positive bacteria, mycobacteria have a thick peptidoglycan layer and lack a true outer membrane. However, their high lipid content often results in poor Gram staining or false-negative reactions. The robust lipid barrier and dense structural integrity impede the diffusion of hydrophilic antibiotics, such as rifampicin, macrolides, fluoroquinolones, and tetracyclines [9].

Many enzymatic systems maintain the integrity of the cell wall, with the biosynthesis of mycolic acids, arabinose, and peptidoglycan being the three primary pathways. The complete and normal expression of the involved genes is crucial for preserving the impermeability of the cell wall and resisting the entry of hydrophilic drugs. Current research in mycobacterial cell wall structure and key enzymes in cell wall synthesis has made exciting progress [10]. Many drugs targeting cell wall synthesis have been developed or are undergoing research, including isoniazid [11], ethionamide [12], and TLM [13, 14] that inhibit mycolic acid synthesis; ethambutol [15], pretomanid, delamanid [16], SQ109 [17], TBA7371 [18–20], OPC-167832 [19, 21], BTZ043 [22, 23], and PBTZ169 [24, 25] that target arabinogalactan synthesis. Conventional β-lactam antibiotics, aimed at peptidoglycan synthesis, exhibit limited efficacy against *M. tuberculosis*, not only due to the production of broad-spectrum β-lactamases but also because of the D, D-transpeptidase enzyme. The mycobacterial cell wall follows an L, D-transpeptidation mode, which does not perfectly align with the target D, D-transpeptidase, thus bringing about a certain degree of intrinsic resistance [26]. It is worth noting that some drugs involved in the cell wall synthesis pathway can simultaneously target other pathways *in vivo*. For instance, pretomanid and delamanid exhibit bactericidal activity against both replicating and non-replicating mycobacteria by affecting multiple essential pathways [27].

In mycobacteria, the abundant lipids provide cellular protection and significantly influence the permeability of small hydrophilic compounds, such as antibiotics. While channel proteins typically facilitate the transport of these compounds across the bacterial outer membrane, most mycobacteria lack such proteins. The only recognized channel protein is MspA, found in fast-growing mycobacteria such as *Mycobacterium smegmatis* [28]. Additionally, molecules are considered to function as channel proteins, such as CpnT, encoded by the *Rv3903c* gene in *M. tuberculosis*, but the knowledge of its role in the transport of hydrophilic compounds remains limited [29].

NTMs such as *Mycobacterium abscessus*, *Mycobacterium avium*, and *Mycobacterium kansasii* frequently exhibit two distinct colony morphologies: smooth and rough. The smooth colonies are uniform, circular, and glossy, while the rough colonies are irregular and dry. *M. avium* and *Mycobacterium intracellulare* can also form smooth opaque or smooth translucent colonies [30–32]. Rough-type variations usually prevail in severe and chronic clinical infections. The transformation mainly depends on the presence of glycopeptidolipids (GPL). For instance, in *M. kansasii*, the smooth phenotype is associated with surface GPL oligomers. The smooth phenotype of *Mycobacterium vaccae* is linked to the presence of complex polyesters. In M. *abscessus*, the transition from smooth to rough is closely related to the reduction of GPL in the outer membrane, which enhances the hydrophobicity of *M. abscessus*, thereby diminishing its susceptibility to hydrophilic antibiotics such as β-lactams, isoniazid, and streptomycin [33, 34]. Rough-type variations confer increased tolerance to antibiotics and facilitate the formation of biofilm structures.

2.2 Drug efflux pumps

Efflux pumps play a crucial role in the inherent drug resistance mechanisms of bacteria, lowering the effective concentration of antibiotics inside the cell and thereby enhancing bacterial tolerance to drugs. Sub-lethal concentrations of antibiotics can stimulate the overexpression and increased activity of existing efflux pumps, promoting the selection of resistant mutants and providing a foundation for high-level resistance. Bacterial efflux pumps are classified into five superfamilies based on sequence homology: (i) the multidrug and toxic compound extrusion (MATE) superfamily, (ii) the resistance nodulation cell division (RND) superfamily, (iii) the small multidrug resistance (SMR) superfamily, (iv) the major facilitator superfamily (MFS), and (v) the ATP-binding cassette (ABC) superfamily. The first four families are classified as secondary transport proteins, where drug efflux is coupled with proton influx. Members of the ABC superfamily are primary transport proteins. They utilize energy derived from the hydrolysis of ATP to transport the drugs across the membrane, contributing the most to antibiotic tolerance in mycobacteria [35]. The genome of *M. tuberculosis* encodes genes for all five efflux pump superfamilies, including many ABC and MFS superfamily proteins. Efflux pumps are often associated with multidrug resistance in mycobacteria, as the same pump could excrete multiple substrates [36]. We summarized the known efflux pumps, their corresponding genes, and substrates in **Table 1**. The efflux pumps in NTM also play pivotal roles in the excretion of antibiotics. The MmpS-MmpL efflux pump system in the *M. abscessus* complex is implicated in the resistance to both clofazimine and bedaquiline [66]. Whole-genome sequencing of the *M. abscessus* complex has revealed that it can encode efflux pumps from all known superfamilies. Currently, in *M. avium*, there has been in-depth research on the MFS superfamily member MAV_1406 and the ABC superfamily members MAV_1695 and MAV_3306, which are responsible for transporting macrolide antibiotics [47, 60]. The LfrA of the MFS superfamily expels fluoroquinolones, ethidium bromide, acridine yellow, dodecyl dimethyl ammonium bromide, and Tet(V), which is involved in tetracycline efflux. The Tap pump in *M. smegmatis*

Superfamily	Locus tag/pump	Known substrates	Strains
ABC	Rv0194 [37]	BL, CHL, EMB, EtBr, MAC, NOV, STR, TET, VAN.	*M. tuberculosis*
	Rv0933/PstB [38]	EMB, FQ, INH, RIF	*M. tuberculosis*
	Rv1217c/18c [39]	BL, INH, RIF, NOV	*M. tuberculosis*
	Rv1456c/57c/58c [40]	EMB, INH, RIF, STR.	M. tuberculosis
	Rv1473 [41, 42]	MAC	*M. tuberculosis*
	Rv1667c/68c [43]	MAC, PZA	*M. tuberculosis*
	Rv1686c/87c [44]	MAC	*M. tuberculosis*
	Rv1819c/BacA [45]	AG, AP, BL, CHL, INH, MAC, NOV, RIF, TET, VAN	*M. tuberculosis*
	Rv2477c [45]	FQ, MAC	*M. tuberculosis*
	Rv2686c/87c/88c [45]	FQ	*M. tuberculosis*
	Rv2936/37/38/Drr [46]	AG, CHL, DAU, DOX, EMB, EtBr, MAC, NOR, PUR, RIF, TET	*M. tuberculosis*
	Rv3756c [43]	PZA	*M. tuberculosis*
	MAV_1695, MAV_3306 [47]	MAC	*M. avium*
	MSMEG_5779/PstB [48]	FQs	*M. smegmatis*

Superfamily	Locus tag/pump	Known substrates	Strains
MFS	Rv0037c [49]	RIF	*M. tuberculosis*
	Rv0191 [43]	RIF, PZA	*M. tuberculosis*
	Rv0783c/EmrB [50]	INH, RIF	*M. tuberculosis*
	Rv0842 [49]	RIF	*M. tuberculosis*
	Rv0849 [49, 51]	BL, INH, RIF	*M. tuberculosis*
	Rv1250 [49]	INH, RIF	*M. tuberculosis*
	Rv1258c/Tap [37, 52]	CFZ, EMB, ERY, EtBr, FQ, INH, RIF, SPE, TET	*M. tuberculosis*
	Rv1410c/P55 [49]	AG, CFZ, INH, RIF, TET	*M. tuberculosis*
	Rv1634 [53]	FQ, INH, RIF	*M. tuberculosis*
	Rv1877 [53, 54]	ACR, ERY, EtBr, INH, KAN, RIF, TET	*M. tuberculosis*
	Rv2209 [45, 49]	OFX, RIF	*M. tuberculosis*
	Rv2265 [49, 53]	INH, RIF	*M. tuberculosis*
	Rv2333c/Stp [49]	RIF, SPE, TET	*M. tuberculosis*
	Rv2456c [49, 53]	INH, RIF	*M. tuberculosis*
	Rv2459/JefA [45, 53]	EMB, EtBr, INH, RIF	*M. tuberculosis*
	Rv2846c/EfpA [45, 55, 56]	ACR, ERY, EtBr, FQ, INH, RIF	*M. tuberculosis*
	Rv3239c [53]	INH, RIF	*M. tuberculosis*
	Rv3728 [45]	EMB, INH, RIF	*M. tuberculosis*
	MAV_1406 [57]	MAC	*M. avium*
	ML0556c/P55 [58–60]	AG, TET	*M. leprae*
	Tap [61]	AG, TET	*M. smegmatis*
	LfrA [62]	FQs, ACR, EtBr, CTAB	*M. smegmatis*
	MSMEG_5187/Tet(V) [61]	TET	*M. smegmatis*
MATE	Rv2836c/DinF	AG, SD	*M. tuberculosis*
	MSMEG_2631 [63]	PLM, BLM, CAP, AMK, KM, CPC	*M. smegmatis*
RND	Rv0676c/MmpL5 [64]	BDQ, CFZ, TET	*M. tuberculosis*
	Rv2942 [65]	BDQ, INH	*M. tuberculosis*
SMR	Rv3065/Mmr [66]	ACR, EtBr, FQ, INH, MAC	*M. tuberculosis*
	MmpS-MmpL [67]	CFZ, BDQ	*M. abscessus*

Note. The drug acronyms included in this table refer to ACR (acridine yellow), AG (aminoglycosides), AP (antimicrobial peptides), BDQ (bedaquiline), BL (β-lactams), CCCP (carbonyl cyanide m-chlorophenyl hydrazone), CFZ (clarithromycin), CHL (chloramphenicol), EMB (ethambutol), ERY (erythromycin), EtBr (ethidium bromide), FQ (fluoroquinolones), INH (isoniazid), MAC (macrolides), NOV (neomycin), PIP (piperine), QRC (quercetin), RES (reserpine), RIF (rifampicin), SPE (spectinomycin), TET (tetracycline), TTD (tetramethylammonium), TZ (thiolactone), VAN (vancomycin), VER (verapamil), PLM (phleomycin), BLM (bleomycin), CAP (capreomycin), and CPC (cetylpyridinium chloride).

Table 1.
Mycobacterium efflux pumps implicated in drug resistance.

also expels aminoglycosides and tetracycline, while the P55 pump contributes to the same in *Mycobacterium leprae*. Notably, MAV_1406 is an efflux pump in *M. avium* that expels clarithromycin [60]. The PstB pump in *M. smegmatis*, belonging to the ABC superfamily, is responsible for transporting fluoroquinolones [48].

2.3 Metabolism slowdown and shifting

Most antibiotics preferentially kill or inhibit metabolically active bacteria. Mycobacteria grow slowly, particularly slow-growing species like *M. tuberculosis*, which divides every 20 hours compared to the typical 20 minutes for *Escherichia coli*. Under antibiotic pressure, mycobacteria undergo metabolic adaptations through regulating interconnected pathways to control energy, carbon, and lipid metabolism, which reduces metabolic and growth rates, extending replication times to over 100 hours [67]. Gene expression related to the tricarboxylic acid (TCA) cycle, aerobic respiration, and ATP synthesis is downregulated, along with the expression of essential components such as 16S RNA and ribosomal protein-coding genes [68].

M. tuberculosis exhibits significant metabolic flexibility; various bypass pathways complicate the resistance situation of drugs. The energy metabolism of *M. tuberculosis* shifts to storage pathways, leading to changes in lipid and redox metabolism following drug exposure. Under various restrictive conditions, cellular carbon fluxes redirect from the tricarboxylic acid cycle (TCA) to carbon storage in fatty acids *via* the triacylglycerol acid cycle (TGA). This redirection is facilitated by the upregulation of the *tgs1* gene, thereby allowing the bacteria to maintain chronic infection at the expense of slowing down their metabolism [69]. Lactic acid and pyruvate can be recycled through gluconeogenesis, valine metabolism, Krebs cycle, GABA shunt, glyoxylic acid shunt, and methyl citrate [70]. When the host cell membrane constitutes the exclusive carbon and energy source, protracted metabolic growth can be upheld through the specialized cholesterol uptake system encoded by the *mce4* gene cluster [71]. It was also reported that isocitrate lyase (ICL) and malate synthase (MS) are identified key targets in bypass pathways, which are safe drug targets since glyoxylate bypass is absent in mammals [72].

The latent infections enhance the survival of mycobacteria under antibiotic treatment [73], with most current drug regimens primarily targeting active bacteria, resulting in limited treatment options. This necessitates prolonged therapy, long-term medication, and hepatotoxicity. Following it always results in poor patient compliance and suboptimal treatment outcomes [74].

The balance between *M. tuberculosis* and host microenvironment resistance can lead to complex granulomatous immune structures, isolating infections to limit bacterial spread, but this isolation also aids pathogens in evading host immune responses and antibiotic effects [75]. *M. tuberculosis* can develop biofilms at the granuloma's periphery near T and B lymphocytes. This not only hinders the infiltration of anti-TB agents, such as isoniazid and rifampicin, but also obstructs the recruitment of immune cells [76–78]. Biofilm formation contributes to relative antibiotic resistance, often manifesting as phenotypic tolerance. Various mycobacterial species have been discovered to form drug-resistant biofilms and often shown to be more resistant to conventional antibiotic treatment, including *M. abscessus*, *M. smegmatis*, *M. avium*, *Mycobacterium fortuitum*, and *Mycobacterium ulcerans* [79–83].

2.4 Degradation and modification of drugs

Upon entering bacterial cells, anti-mycobacterial agents encounter numerous challenges to exert their intended effects. The diverse enzymes were reported to degrade and modify the drugs. Early studies on penicillin have indicated that *M. tuberculosis* possesses inherent resistance to this antibiotic due to the expression of β-lactamase

[84, 85]. *M. tuberculosis* genome encodes for class A β-lactamase and BlaC, which exhibits broad substrate specificity [86]. Nevertheless, in clinical settings, this form of drug degradation can be inhibited by the β-lactamase inhibitor clavulanic acid [87].

The acetylation, ribosylation, and methylation were reported to modify the anti-mycobacterial drugs. The *eis* gene in *M. tuberculosis* encodes an acetyltransferase that can acetylate aminoglycoside antibiotics such as kanamycin A and cyclic peptide antibiotics such as capreomycin, thereby inactivating them [88, 89]. Mutations in several promoters and the transcriptional regulator whiB7 can lead to the overexpression of *eis*, conferring a low level of resistance to kanamycin A [88, 90]. The *arr* gene (*MAB_0591*) encodes an ADP-ribosyltransferase that catalyzes the ADP-ribosylation of rifampicin, rendering it inactive [91]. Ribosylative inactivation of rifampin was also observed in *M. smegmatis* [92–94]. Recently, discovered pyridine-benzimidazole compounds have emerged as novel anti-TB agents, serving as nanomolar inhibitors of the enzyme DprE1 essential for synthesizing arabinogalactan. However, these compounds can be N-methylated by the methyltransferase encoded by the *Rv0560c* gene in *M. tuberculosis*, causing a loss of their inhibitory effects [95].

2.5 Target modification and mimicry

The natural resistance mechanism of mycobacteria to antimicrobial agents manifests in the inactivation of the drugs themselves and modifications of drug targets. Macrolide antibiotics inhibit bacterial ribosomes by binding to the 50S ribosomal subunit. *M. tuberculosis* encodes the methyltransferase Erm (37), which monomethylates the 2057–2059 residues of 23S rRNA, thereby conferring tolerance to macrolides [96, 97]. Other mycobacterial species express homologous enzymes, such as Erm (38) in *M. smegmatis* and Erm (39) in *M. fortuitum* [98, 99]. It is worth noting that all mycobacterial erm genes are inducible. For example, most strains of *M. abscessus* harbor erm (41), and exposure to macrolide drugs can induce their overexpression, thus elevating resistance levels [100].

Rifampicin primarily exerts its bactericidal effect by interfering with the transcriptional function of RNA polymerase. Mycobacteria can encode RNA polymerase-binding protein RbpA, a specific transcriptional activator that regulates rifampicin binding to RNA polymerase. This modulation increases the resistance of mycobacteria to rifampicin and can underlie high-level resistance [101]. Mutations in the ethambutol resistance determination region (ERDR) within the arabinosyl transferase *embB* gene in *M. tuberculosis* led to drug resistance, and it is noteworthy that *M. abscessus* naturally possesses the same mutations in the *embB* gene, thereby it inherently resists ethambutol [102].

In addition to directly modifying the targets, mycobacteria can also encode analogs of these targets, achieving drug tolerance through competitive binding. Fluoroquinolones target the mycobacterial DNA gyrase-DNA complex. The disruption of gyrase activity leads to DNA breakage. Both M. *tuberculosis* and *M. smegmatis* can encode pentapeptide repeat proteins (PRPs) named MfpA, which possess a similar structure and charge as double-stranded DNA. These proteins reversibly bind to the GyrB subunit of the DNA gyrase, inhibiting its enzymatic activity and reducing the entry of normal DNA into the drug-mediated DNA breakage pathway. Conversely, MfpA binds to the ATPase domain of gyrase and activates the ATP hydrolysis activity, which facilitates the release of fluoroquinolone drugs from the DNA gyrase-drug-DNA complex [103, 104].

3. Acquired resistance mechanism

Mycobacteria predominantly develop acquired resistance primarily through point mutations in contrast to the ESKAPE bacteria (*Enterococcus faecium*, *Staphylococcus aureus*, *Klebsiella pneumonia*, *Acinetobacter baumannii*, *Pseudomonas aeruginosa*, and *Enterobacter species*), which primarily acquire resistance through extensive horizontal gene transfer (HGT). In these acquired resistance mechanisms of mycobacteria, the overexpression of drug targets and efflux pumps results in low-level resistance, while high-level resistance is generally attributed to mutations in target genes and the failure of prodrug activation [3–5, 79].

3.1 Overdose of drug target

In response to the stimulus of antibiotics, bacteria may generate promoter mutations that lead to the overexpression of drug targets. For instance, both ethambutol and D-cycloserine can induce low-level resistance due to an excess of their respective targets [105].

Ethambutol acts as a structural analog of decaprenyl-monophosphoryl-D-arabinose (DPA), competing with DPA for binding to arabinosyl transferase, thus hindering cell wall synthesis and resulting in bacterial death [106]. Mutations in the *Rv3806c* gene, which encodes the phosphoribosyl transferase UbiA, represent one of the bacterial strategies for countering ethambutol. UbiA mediates the synthesis of the cell wall precursor 5-phospho-α-ribosyl-1-pyrophosphate (PRPP) and is a key enzyme in the DPA synthesis pathway. Mutations in *Rv3806c* increase intracellular levels of DPA, thereby competitively inhibiting the binding of ethambutol to arabinosyl transferase, which cause observable ethambutol resistance [105].

Alanine racemase (encoded by *Rv3423c/alr*) and D-alanine ligase (encoded by *Rv2981/ddlA*) serve as essential catalytic enzymes in the synthesis of peptidoglycan precursors in the mycobacterial cell wall [107, 108]. D-cycloserine suppresses peptidoglycan synthesis by competitively inhibiting these two enzymes, and mutations resulting in overexpression can confer resistance to D-cycloserine in both *M. tuberculosis* and *M. smegmatis* [109–111]. Additionally, reports have indicated that the overexpression of inhA, the prime target of isoniazid and ethionamide, can also lead to low-level resistance in *M. smegmatis*, *M. bovis* BCG, and *M. tuberculosis* [112, 113].

3.2 Mutations in the efflux pump system and correlated regulatory factor

Efflux pumps play an important role in intrinsic resistance and contribute to higher-level resistance through gene mutations that encode efflux pumps or regulate their transcription. Those mutations may lead to efflux pump overexpression in response to antibiotic pressure. The *iniA* gene (*Rv0342*) in *M. tuberculosis* encodes an efflux pump responsible for transporting isoniazid and ethambutol; mutations in this gene are associated with moderate- to low-level multidrug tolerance [114]. Additionally, mutations in the transcriptional regulator *Rv0678* lead to the overexpression of the multidrug efflux pump MmpL5, resulting in cross-resistance of the bacteria to clofazimine and bedaquiline [115, 116]. Furthermore, mutations in the transcriptional TetR repressor *MAB_4384*, which regulates the expression of the MmpS5-MmpL5 efflux pump in *M. abscesses*, confer resistance to various thiazole analogs [117, 118].

3.3 Mutations in target and correlated regulatory factor

In acquired resistance in mycobacteria, mutations in drug targets are regarded as the most common mechanism. This acquired resistance involves the resistance to a wide array of antituberculosis agents and antibiotics, encompassing multiple first-line antituberculosis drugs and commonly utilized second-line agents, including rifampicin, isoniazid, ethambutol, streptomycin, bedaquiline, linezolid, fluoroquinolones, amikacin, and kanamycin. The emergence of such resistance poses a substantial challenge to clinical treatment.

Resistance to rifampin in mycobacteria is primarily attributable to mutations in the *rpoB* gene. Rifampicin exerts its effects by binding with high affinity to the β subunit of DNA-dependent RNA polymerase (RpoB), subsequently inhibiting the transcriptional capabilities of mycobacteria [119]. Specifically, mutations occurring within the rifampicin resistance-determining region (RRDR) of the *rpoB* gene (comprising an 81 base pair sequence) diminish its affinity for rifampicin [119, 120].

Isoniazid primarily targets the NADH-dependent enoyl-acyl carrier protein reductase InhA. Mutations in both the structural gene and promoter regions of InhA can lead to resistance against isoniazid [121]. Identified mutations include frameshift insertions, partial gene deletions, missense mutations, and amino acid replacements [122].

The *rpsL*, *rrs*, and *gidB* genes encode S12, 16S rRNA, and glucose inhibition division protein B of protein synthesis apparatus in mycobacterial organisms, respectively. Streptomycin inhibits protein synthesis through its irreversible binding to the ribosomal protein S12 and 16S rRNA. Genetic mutations occurring in these loci lead to the development of streptomycin resistance [123, 124].

Ethambutol is a structural analog of decaprenylmonophosphoryl-D-arabinose (DPA). The primary mechanism of acquired resistance to ethambutol involves inhibiting the arabinosyl transferase activity associated with the EmbCAB protein, which is integral to the biosynthesis of arabinose in the cell wall [125, 126]. The *embCAB* gene encodes this enzyme and consists of three consecutive genes: *embB*, *embA*, and *embC*. In M. *tuberculosis* isolates, resistance to ethambutol has been linked to chromosomal mutations within the *embB* gene primarily, which are concentrated in a 576-bp segment known as the ethambutol resistance-determining region (ERDR). A series of codon mutations within ERDR were exploited in EMB-resistant mycobacteria, with codon variations of *embB* at 306, 406, and 497 positions identified as hotspots for mutations [127, 128].

Mycobacteria possess an intrinsic mechanism that modifies target sites, resulting in natural resistance to corresponding drugs. Furthermore, mutations in the genes associated with this mechanism can lead to an enhanced level of drug resistance. Fluoroquinolones target the gyrase enzymes involved in the DNA replication process of mycobacteria. This enzyme consists of two subunits of GyrA and two of GyrB, encoded by the *gyrA* and *gyrB* genes [129]. In contrast to the inherent tolerance caused by the expression of MfpA, acquired resistance in *M. tuberculosis* to fluoroquinolones predominantly results from point mutations within the quinolone resistance-determining region (QRDR) of *gyrA*, followed by mutations in *gyrB*. The GyrA and GyrB mutations diminish the fluoroquinolone binding affinity but would not affect the replication of the mycobacterial DNA. These mutations culminate in high-level resistance, as the gyrase is mycobacteria's sole target of fluoroquinolones [130, 131]. Fluoroquinolones are extensively utilized to treat various infections and serve as the most effective second-line agents against MDR tuberculosis. The emergence of fluoroquinolones resistance *M. tuberculosis* strains compels us to reassess and modify anti-TB treatment strategies accordingly.

The *rrs* genes encode 16S rRNA. Aminoglycoside antibiotics, such as kanamycin, amikacin, and enviomycin, alongside peptide-based drugs such as capreomycin and viomycin, inhibit protein synthesis in mycobacteria by disrupting the function of 16S rRNA. The identified resistance of aminoglycoside and peptide-based drugs is largely associated with mutations of *rrs* genes in *M. tuberculosis, M. abscessus*, and *M. avium* [132–134]. The A1401G, C1402T, and G1484T point mutations within *rrs* in *M. tuberculosis* are responsible for high-level resistance to amikacin and kanamycin [135]. Furthermore, mutations in the *tylA* gene, which encodes the rRNA methyltransferase and 2'-O-methylates in 16S and 23S rRNAs, can also confer resistance to capreomycin and viomycin in *M. tuberculosis* [136].

Linezolid is approved for the treatment of XDR-TB and treatment-intolerant or nonresponsive MDR-TB. It acts on the 50S ribosomal subunit, specifically, the peptidyl-transferase center (PTC), thus blocking tRNA binding and inhibiting ribosomal protein synthesis [137, 138]. Mutations in the PTC of *rrl* gene (encoded 23S rRNA) confer linezolid resistance [139–141]. Additionally, mutations in the *rplC* gene (encoded ribosomal L3 protein) have been identified as resistant to linezolid, both *in vitro* generated or clinically isolated mycobacteria. The most common mutation of *rplC* is T460C [142].

3.4 Abolition of prodrug activation

Prodrugs require activation within the bacterial microenvironment to manifest their therapeutic efficacy. Many anti-TB pharmaceuticals and antibiotics are reported prodrugs, including isoniazid, pyrazinamide, ethionamide, p-aminosalicylic acid, delamanid, and pretomanid [143]. The catalase-peroxidase (KatG), ethionamide-activating enzyme (EthA), pyrazinamidase (PZase), dihydrofolate synthetase (DHPS), dihydrofolate reductase (DHFS), and deazaflavin (F_{420})-dependent nitroreductase (Ddn) are prodrug activation enzymes in mycobacteria.

Isoniazid necessitates activation by KatG, whose primary target is the NADH-dependent enoyl-acyl carrier protein reductase InhA [144, 145]. Mutations occurring in the structural genes or promoters of KatG can result in activation failure, thereby hindering isoniazid from interacting with NADH/NAD+ to form INH-NAD adducts. Ethylthioisonicamide is the structural analog of isoniazid. Acquired resistance to this prodrug is also associated with these mutations of KatG [146]. Additionally, mutations in the structural genes or promoters of InhA may also confer resistance to isoniazid, [121] as previously mentioned in Section 3.3 of this chapter.

EthA (encoded by gene *Rv3854c*) is an NADPH-specific flavin adenine dinucleotide (FAD) monooxygenase that activates the second-line drug ethionamide (ETH). The EthA monooxygenase activates ETH to an active form. Activated ETH interacts with NAD+ to form an ETH-NAD adduct, which hampers the activity of InhA reductase. The point mutation of *Rv3854c* (G604C) in *M. tuberculosis* has been reported to modulate ETH activation and lead to ETH resistance [12, 113, 147]. Thiacetazone (TAC) was previously used in conjunction with isoniazid to treat MDR-TB. S-oxidation on the thioamide moiety is necessary for the TAC activation. Mutations in EthA can confer TAC resistance in the mycobacteria [117, 148].

PZase/nicotinamidase, encoded by the *pncA* gene in *M. tuberculosis*, catalyzes the conversion of pyrazinamide into its active form, pyrazinoic acid (POA). PZA is a first-line TB drug that targets multiple processes, including energy production, trans-translation, and possibly the pantothenate/coenzyme A pathway. The activity of PZA increases along with decrease in metabolic activity, enabling it to uniquely inhibit semi-dormant bacilli that persist in acidic environments. Mutations in the *pncA* gene, which are highly diverse and scatter along the gene, cause pyrazinamide resistance in mycobacteria [149–151].

DHPS and DHFS are encoded by *folP1* and *folC* genes in mycobacteria. Both DHPS and DHFS are the key essential enzymes in folate biosynthesis. Para-aminosalicylic acid (PAS) is a prodrug activated by DHPS and DHFS enzymes in the folate synthesis pathway to produce hydroxyfolate-like compounds that compete with folate metabolism downstream targets [146]. Mutations within the coding sequence of the dihydropteroate-binding pocket of the *folC* gene would cause failure of prodrug activation, conferring resistance to PAS in mycobacteria as found in clinical isolates [152, 153].

Ddn, encoded by the *ddn* gene in mycobacteria, transforms delamanid and pretomanid into active derivatives. Active forms of these two nitroimidazole compounds target the synthesis of arabinogalactan in the mycobacterial cell wall, specifically inhibiting decaprenylphosphoryl-2-keto-β-D-erythro-pentose reductase (DprE2), which catalyzes the reduction of decaprenylphosphoryl-2-ketoribose (DPX) into decaprenylphosphoryl-D-arabinose (DPA) [16]. Acquired resistance is primarily associated with mutations in the *ddn* gene. Mutations in essential genes involved in the biosynthesis and recycling the F_{420} cofactor, such as *fgd1*, *fbiA*, *fbiB*, and *fbiC*, can also lead to delamanid and pretomanid resistance. Identified mutations include non-synonymous SNPs, small indels, large deletions, and mutations in the promoter region [154–156]. The mechanisms of these two drugs killing mycobacteria likely involve multiple pathways and have not yet been clearly defined. *Rv0077c* may be involved in the metabolism of delamanid and pretomanid intermediates; mutations in the transcriptional repressor (encoded by *Rv0078*) of *Rv0077c* lead to increased expression of *Rv0077c*, thereby reducing the amount of active nitroimidazole compounds, and exhibited the delamanid and pretomanid resistance [157].

Notably, the prodrug-activating enzymes are not essential for the growth and viability of mycobacteria. Mutations, insertions/deletions, and the insertion of mobile genetic elements can disrupt genes encoding prodrug activators without adversely affecting bacterial survival. Moreover, mutations in gene promoters may decrease transcription levels, subsequently lowering the availability of enzymes responsible for prodrug activation.

4. Overcoming drug resistance

In recent years, research on the mechanisms of mycobacterial resistance has enhanced clinical diagnostic and therapeutic capabilities. The conventional approach to preventing drug resistance typically involves the combination of antibiotics in hopes of increasing successful treatment. A fully oral regimen consisting of bedaquiline, pretomanid, linezolid, and moxifloxacin has been clinically validated to partially overcome drug resistance [158–162]. However, both first- and second-line anti-TB drugs included in current treatment regimens have exhibited resistance. Bedaquiline, pretomanid, and delamanid, which were introduced within the last decade for the treatment of MDR-TB, have also exhibited resistance [163]. Drug-resistant tuberculosis remains a significant global health challenge.

The existing drugs fail to meet clinical needs, prompting ongoing research and development of new anti-TB agents. This includes the exploration of the anti-mycobacterial potential of drugs from other therapeutic areas, the investigation of natural products for their anti-mycobacterial properties, and the research of candidate drugs with novel mechanisms. Potential drug target discovery encompasses deep digging into key enzymes involved in the synthesis pathways of cell walls, DNA replication, protein synthesis, and energy metabolism pathways. The anti-TB drug candidate pipeline is promising [164, 165].

The development of novel drugs with innovative mechanisms represents a primary strategy for addressing the challenges posed by existing drug resistance. An exemplary drug exhibiting a new mechanism against tuberculosis is cholesterol catabolism inhibitor GSK2556286 (GSK286). This drug functions *via* Rv1625c, a membrane-bound adenylyl cyclase found in *M. tuberculosis*, and is currently undergoing clinical trials (Phase IIa) for systemic application in the treatment of tuberculosis [166]. Compound GSK3036656 (ganfeborole) targets and inhibits the leucyl-tRNA synthetase LeuRS of the protein synthesis pathway. Currently, it is undergoing an open-label, randomized trial (Phase IIa) [165]. Other emerging targets include cytochrome bd in the respiratory chain, cytidine triphosphate synthetase PyrG, HsaD in the cholesterol catabolic pathway, tryptophan synthase TrpAB, fumarate hydratase in the tricarboxylic acid cycle, iron-dependent regulator protein IdeR, and novel targets in host-directed therapies (HDTs). Those targets have significant potential in the fight against drug-resistant tuberculosis and underlining further verification and refinement [164].

In new drug development, synthesizing novel compounds is often time-consuming and costly; therefore, drug repurposing and utilizing natural products may be economical alternatives. An illustrative example of repurposing an existing drug is represented by the class of azole antifungal agents, which are structural analogs of linezolid. The administration of linezolid has been associated with significant adverse effects, notably myelosuppression and serotonergic toxicity, which can culminate in a potentially life-threatening condition known as serotonin syndrome [167, 168]. In recent years, linezolid-tolerant mycobacterial strains have emerged. The structural architecture of azole antifungal drugs resembles that of linezolid, positioning them as promising candidates for the treatment of tuberculosis. Notably, four azole antifungal agents, posaconazole, itraconazole, miconazole, and clotrimazole, have demonstrated anti-mycobacterial potency and good efficacy against MDR-TB clinical isolates [169]. Another example is the repurposing of terlipressin (glypressin) to treat ethambutol-resistant mycobacteria. Mutations in EmbC, the key enzyme involved in the biosynthesis of arabinogalactan and lipoarabinomannan, confer resistance to ethambutol. A drug screening study conducted on the FDA inventory identified terlipressin possessed a greater binding affinity for EmbC than ethambutol, suggesting its potential as an alternative treatment in cases of ethambutol resistance [170].

Natural compounds with anti-mycobacterial activity encompass a diverse range of classes, including lipids and fatty acids, simple aromatic compounds, phenolics and quinones, peptides, alkaloids, terpenes, steroids, and various other structures, sourced extensively from plants, bacteria, fungi, and marine organisms [171–174]. Naphthoquinones isolated from *Diospyros anisandra* exhibited potent activity against drug-resistant *M. tuberculosis* strains [175]. Flavanone pinocembrin (dihydrochrysin) and biochanin A demonstrated EtBr efflux inhibitory activity comparable to reference efflux pump inhibitors (EPIs) [176, 177]. Other natural products that exhibit promising activity in the fight against drug-resistant *M. tuberculosis* infections include thiolactomycin, pyridomycin, novobiocin, lipiarmycin A3, gladiolin, and kanglemycin A, (S)-(−)-acidomycin, ecumicin, lassomycin, and cyclomarin A, most of which are cyclic peptides [178]. *Scutellaria baicalensis* extract inhibits planktonic *M. abscessus* growth and reduces the bacterial adhesion and aggregation of *M. abscessus* biofilm formation [179]. Marine-derived fungal sesterterpenes and ophiobolins inhibit the biofilm formation of *M. bovis* BCG and *M. smegmatis* [180]. Due to the generally low yield of natural compounds, coupled with their relatively high structural complexity, significant attention is being paid to research endeavors. Natural compounds not only exhibit antimicrobial properties but also demonstrate resistance-inhibiting effects. They continue to hold great value for novel drug development [162, 181].

Bacteriophages typically exhibit a lower propensity to induce resistance and target a specific spectrum of bacterial strains [182]. Their host specificity reduces potential harm to normal microbiota in the host, yet it also complicates the selection of effective phages [183]. Bacteriophages represent an alternative therapeutic option, especially in the treatment of *M. abscessus* infections, and strains with rough morphology are completely resistant to antimicrobial agents [184, 185]. Mycobacteriophages have now been recognized for their therapeutic value in the context of rising drug-resistant infections [186]. Extensive research has demonstrated that mycobacteriophage cocktails can reduce bacterial burden in patients with cystic fibrosis and mitigate the risk of infection following lung transplantation [162, 187, 188]. Consequently, phage therapy has emerged as one of the most promising alternative treatments.

The increasing availability of candidate drugs, clinically approved medications, and the implementation of phage therapies significantly advanced the therapeutic options for drug-resistant mycobacteria. These therapies are specifically tailored to address infection sites and resistance phenotypes and may help to improve the treatment of drug-resistant mycobacteria [189].

5. Conclusion

Mycobacteria possess a high lipid content cell wall, which impedes the penetration of drugs. The bacteria encode multiple enzymes taking responsibility for decreasing the drug concentration, for example, efflux, degrade, or modify the target drugs. Mycobacteria can alter their metabolic pathways or modify drug targets in response to drug treatment. Collectively, these factors contribute to the complex mechanisms of the mycobacterial inherent resistance. On the other hand, mycobacteria can develop formidable acquired resistance through genetic mutations occurring at drug targets, efflux pumps, and prodrug-activating enzymes. Those genetic mutations in target genes and the failure of prodrug activation often led to high-level resistance.

Mycobacteriophages exhibited therapeutic value in the context of rising drug-resistant infections; however, there is a possibility that phages may carry virulence genes, and their immunogenicity remains a significant concern. The formulation of antibiotic combination regimens may enhance patient adherence by increasing drug dosages and shortening treatment durations. Currently, the treatment of drug-resistant mycobacterial infections involves the introduction of new anti-TB drugs, alongside the formulation of combination regimens. Nevertheless, in light of the dynamic inherent and acquired resistance mechanisms, these strategies often prove inadequate in the face of mycobacteria resistance.

A primary strategy to address drug-resistant challenges is to develop innovative novel mechanism drugs. Additionally, drug repurposing and the exploration of natural products represent promising prospects. The resistance mechanisms of mycobacteria remain a global focus, with a series of new emerging anti-mycobacteria drugs currently under the development or in clinical trials. In the future, the approved new drugs, new regimens, and new phage therapies hold promise to overcome the existing drug-resistant mycobacteria.

In this chapter, we provide a comprehensive overview of the intrinsic and acquired mechanisms of drug resistance in mycobacteria, along with the strategies and innovative approaches to combat the resistance. Hopefully, this chapter will enhance our understanding of drug-resistant mycobacteria, thereby contributing to developing more effective strategies for combating drug-resistant mycobacteria in the future.

Acknowledgements

This work was supported by the Technological Innovation and Development Project of Chengdu Bureau of Science and Technology (2024-YF05-00039-SN), the National Base for International Science and Technology Cooperation of Chengdu University (ARRLKF23-06), and the Fundamental Research Funds for the Central Universities (YJ201985). Figdraw drew **Figure 1** of this chapter.

Conflict of interest

All authors declare no potential conflicts of interest concerning the authorship and/or publication of this chapter.

Author details

Jumei Zeng[1]*, Xingyan Tan[1] and Chao Gao[2]

1 West China-PUMC C.C. Chen Institute of Health, West China School of Public Health and West China Fourth Hospital, Sichuan University, Chengdu, China

2 Laboratory of Human Diseases and Immunotherapies, West China Hospital, Sichuan University, Chengdu, China

*Address all correspondence to: zengjumei@scu.edu.cn

References

[1] World Health Organization. Global Tuberculosis Report 2023. WHO; 2024. Available from: https://www.who.int/publications/i/item/9789240083851

[2] Shih DC, Cassidy PM, Perkins KM, Crist MB, Cieslak PR, Leman RL. Extrapulmonary nontuberculous mycobacterial disease surveillance - Oregon, 2014-2016. MMWR. Morbidity and Mortality Weekly Report. 2018;**67**(31):854-857. DOI: 10.15585/mmwr.mm6731a3

[3] Nguyen L. Antibiotic resistance mechanisms in *M. tuberculosis*: An update. Archives of Toxicology. 2016;**90**(7):1585-1604. DOI: 10.1007/s00204-016-1727-6

[4] Sachan R, Mistry V, Dholaria M, Rana A, Devgon I, Ali I, et al. Overcoming *Mycobacterium tuberculosis* drug resistance: Novel medications and repositioning strategies. ACS Omega. 2023;**8**(36):32244-32257. DOI: 10.1021/acsomega.3c02563

[5] Li H, Yuan J, Duan S, Pang Y. Resistance and tolerance of *Mycobacterium tuberculosis* to antimicrobial agents-how *M. tuberculosis* can escape antibiotics. WIREs Mechanisms of Disease. 2022;**14**(6):e1573. DOI: 10.1002/wsbm.1573

[6] Brown-Elliott BA, Nash KA, Wallace RJ. Antimicrobial susceptibility testing, drug resistance mechanisms, and therapy of infections with nontuberculous mycobacteria. Clinical Microbiology Reviews. 2012;**25**(3):545-582. DOI: 10.1128/CMR.05030-11

[7] Cole ST, Brosch R, Parkhill J, Garnier T, Churcher C, Harris D, et al. Deciphering the biology of *Mycobacterium tuberculosis* from the complete genome sequence. Nature. 1998;**393**(6685):537-544. DOI: 10.1038/31159

[8] Hett EC, Rubin EJ. Bacterial growth and cell division: A mycobacterial perspective. Microbiology and Molecular Biology Reviews. 2008;**72**(1):126-156. DOI: 10.1128/MMBR.00028-07

[9] Brennan PJ, Nikaido H. The envelope of mycobacteria. Annual Review of Biochemistry. 1995;**64**:29-63. DOI: 10.1146/annurev.bi.64.070195.000333

[10] Xu X, Dong B, Peng L, Gao C, He Z, Wang C, et al. Anti-tuberculosis drug development via targeting the cell envelope of *Mycobacterium tuberculosis*. Frontiers in Microbiology. 2022;**13**:1056608. DOI: 10.3389/fmicb.2022.1056608

[11] Vilcheze C, Jacobs WJ. The isoniazid paradigm of killing, resistance, and persistence in *Mycobacterium tuberculosis*. Journal of Molecular Biology. 2019;**431**(18):3450-3461. DOI: 10.1016/j.jmb.2019.02.016

[12] Vilcheze C, Jacobs WJ. Resistance to isoniazid and ethionamide in *Mycobacterium tuberculosis*: Genes, mutations, and causalities. Microbiology Spectrum. 2014;**2**(4):M2-M14. DOI: 10.1128/Microbiolspec.MGM2-0014-2013

[13] Choi KH, Kremer L, Besra GS, Rock CO. Identification and substrate specificity of beta-ketoacyl (acyl carrier protein) synthase III (mtFabH) from *Mycobacterium tuberculosis*. The Journal of Biological Chemistry.

2000;**275**(36):28201-28207. DOI: 10.1074/jbc.M003241200

[14] Kremer L, Douglas JD, Baulard AR, Morehouse C, Guy MR, Alland D, et al. Thiolactomycin and related analogues as novel anti-mycobacterial agents targeting KasA and KasB condensing enzymes in *Mycobacterium tuberculosis*. The Journal of Biological Chemistry. 2000;**275**(22):16857-16864. DOI: 10.1074/jbc.M000569200

[15] Zhang L, Zhao Y, Gao Y, Wu L, Gao R, Zhang Q, et al. Structures of cell wall arabinosyltransferases with the anti-tuberculosis drug ethambutol. Science. 2020;**368**(6496):1211-1219. DOI: 10.1126/Science.aba9102

[16] Abrahams KA, Batt SM, Gurcha SS, Veerapen N, Bashiri G, Besra GS. DprE2 is a molecular target of the anti-tubercular nitroimidazole compounds pretomanid and delamanid. Nature Communications. 2023;**14**(1):3828. DOI: 10.1038/s41467-023-39300-z

[17] Tahlan K, Wilson R, Kastrinsky DB, Arora K, Nair V, Fischer E, et al. SQ109 targets MmpL3, a membrane transporter of trehalose monomycolate involved in mycolic acid donation to the cell wall core of *Mycobacterium tuberculosis*. Antimicrobial Agents and Chemotherapy. 2012;**56**(4):1797-1809. DOI: 10.1128/AAC.05708-11

[18] Chatterji M, Shandil R, Manjunatha MR, Solapure S, Ramachandran V, Kumar N, et al. 1,4-azaindole, a potential drug candidate for treatment of tuberculosis. Antimicrobial Agents and Chemotherapy. 2014;**58**(9):5325-5331. DOI: 10.1128/AAC.03233-14

[19] Robertson GT, Ramey ME, Massoudi LM, Carter CL, Zimmerman M, Kaya F, et al. Comparative analysis of pharmacodynamics in the C3HeB/FeJ mouse tuberculosis model for DprE1 inhibitors TBA-7371, PBTZ169, and OPC-167832. Antimicrobial Agents and Chemotherapy. 2021;**65**(11):e58321. DOI: 10.1128/AAC.00583-21

[20] Zhang G, Guo S, Cui H, Qi J. Virtual screening of small molecular inhibitors against DprE1. Molecules. 2018;**23**(3):524. DOI: 10.3390/molecules23030524

[21] Hariguchi N, Chen X, Hayashi Y, Kawano Y, Fujiwara M, Matsuba M, et al. OPC-167832, a novel carbostyril derivative with potent antituberculosis activity as a DprE1 inhibitor. Antimicrobial Agents and Chemotherapy. 2020;**64**(6):e02020-19. DOI: 10.1128/AAC.02020-19

[22] Makarov V, Manina G, Mikusova K, Mollmann U, Ryabova O, Saint-Joanis B, et al. Benzothiazinones kill *Mycobacterium tuberculosis* by blocking arabinan synthesis. Science. 2009;**324**(5928):801-804. DOI: 10.1126/Science.1171583

[23] Trefzer C, Rengifo-Gonzalez M, Hinner MJ, Schneider P, Makarov V, Cole ST, et al. Benzothiazinones: Prodrugs that covalently modify the decaprenylphosphoryl-beta-D-ribose 2′-epimerase DprE1 of *Mycobacterium tuberculosis*. Journal of the American Chemical Society. 2010;**132**(39):13663-13665. DOI: 10.1021/ja106357w

[24] Makarov V, Lechartier B, Zhang M, Neres J, van der Sar AM, Raadsen SA, et al. Towards a new combination therapy for tuberculosis with next generation benzothiazinones. EMBO Molecular Medicine. 2014;**6**(3):372-383. DOI: 10.1002/emmm.201303575

[25] Shi J, Lu J, Wen S, Zong Z, Huo F, Luo J, et al. *In vitro* activity of PBTZ169 against multiple *Mycobacterium* species.

Antimicrobial Agents and Chemotherapy. 2018;**62**(11):e01314-e01318. DOI: 10.1128/AAC.01314-18

[26] Gupta R, Lavollay M, Mainardi JL, Arthur M, Bishai WR, Lamichhane G. The *Mycobacterium tuberculosis* protein LdtMt2 is a nonclassical transpeptidase required for virulence and resistance to amoxicillin. Nature Medicine. 2010;**16**(4):466-469. DOI: 10.1038/nm.2120

[27] Singh R, Manjunatha U, Boshoff HI, Ha YH, Niyomrattanakit P, Ledwidge R, et al. PA-824 kills nonreplicating *Mycobacterium tuberculosis* by intraCellular NO release. Science. 2008;**322**(5906):1392-1395. DOI: 10.1126/Science.1164571

[28] Faller M, Niederweis M, Schulz GE. The structure of a mycobacterial outer-membrane channel. Science. 2004;**303**(5661):1189-1192. DOI: 10.1126/Science.1094114

[29] Danilchanka O, Sun J, Pavlenok M, Maueroder C, Speer A, Siroy A, et al. An outer membrane channel protein of *Mycobacterium tuberculosis* with exotoxin activity. Proceedings of the National Academy of Sciences of the United States of America. 2014;**111**(18):6750-6755. DOI: 10.1073/pnas.1400136111

[30] Belisle JT, Brennan PJ. Chemical basis of rough and smooth variation in mycobacteria. Journal of Bacteriology. 1989;**171**(6):3465-3470. DOI: 10.1128/jb.171.6.3465-3470.1989

[31] Bernut A, Viljoen A, Dupont C, Sapriel G, Blaise M, Bouchier C, et al. Insights into the smooth-to-rough transitioning in *Mycobacterium bolletii* unravels a functional Tyr residue conserved in all mycobacterial MmpL family members. Molecular Microbiology. 2016;**99**(5):866-883. DOI: 10.1111/mmi.13283

[32] Prinzis S, Rivoire B, Brennan PJ. Search for the molecular basis of morphological variation in *Mycobacterium avium*. Infection and Immunity. 1994;**62**(5):1946-1951. DOI: 10.1128/iai.62.5.1946-1951.1994

[33] Belisle JT, Klaczkiewicz K, Brennan PJ, Jacobs WJ, Inamine JM. Rough morphological variants of *Mycobacterium avium*. Characterization of genomic deletions resulting in the loss of glycopeptidolipid expression. The Journal of Biological Chemistry. 1993;**268**(14):10517-10523

[34] Parmar S, Tocheva EI. The cell envelope of *Mycobacterium abscessus* and its role in pathogenesis. PLoS Pathogens. 2023;**19**(5):e1011318. DOI: 10.1371/journal.ppat.1011318

[35] De Rossi E, Ainsa JA, Riccardi G. Role of mycobacterial efflux transporters in drug resistance: An unresolved question. FEMS Microbiology Reviews. 2006;**30**(1):36-52. DOI: 10.1111/j.1574-6976.2005.00002.x

[36] Laws M, Jin P, Rahman KM. Efflux pumps in *Mycobacterium tuberculosis* and their inhibition to tackle antimicrobial resistance. Trends in Microbiology. 2022;**30**(1):57-68. DOI: 10.1016/j.tim.2021.05.001

[37] Malinga L, Brand J, Olorunju S, Stoltz A, van der Walt M. Molecular analysis of genetic mutations among cross-resistant second-line injectable drugs reveals a new resistant mutation in *Mycobacterium tuberculosis*. Diagnostic Microbiology and Infectious Disease. 2016;**85**(4):433-437. DOI: 10.1016/j.diagmicrobio.2016.05.010

[38] Lu J, Liu M, Wang Y, Pang Y, Zhao Z. Mechanisms of fluoroquinolone monoresistance in *Mycobacterium tuberculosis*. FEMS Microbiology Letters. 2014;**353**(1):40-48. DOI: 10.1111/1574-6968.12401

[39] Wang K, Pei H, Huang B, Zhu X, Zhang J, Zhou B, et al. The expression of ABC efflux pump, *Rv1217c-Rv1218c*, and its association with multidrug resistance of *Mycobacterium tuberculosis* in China. Current Microbiology. 2013;**66**(3):222-226. DOI: 10.1007/s00284-012-0215-3

[40] Ozgur D, Ersoy L, Ulger M, Tezcan US, Aslan G. Investigation of efflux pump genes in resistant *Mycobacterium tuberculosis* complex clinical isolates exposed to first line antituberculosis drugs and verapamil combination. Mikrobiyoloji Bülteni. 2023;**57**(2):207-219. DOI: 10.5578/mb.20239916

[41] Lee JJ, Kang HY, Lee WI, Cho SY, Kim YJ, Lee HJ. Efflux pump gene expression study using RNA-seq in multidrug-resistant TB. The International Journal of Tuberculosis and Lung Disease. 2021;**25**(12):974-981. DOI: 10.5588/ijtld.21.0117

[42] Duan W, Li X, Ge Y, Yu Z, Li P, Li J, et al. *Mycobacterium tuberculosis Rv1473* is a novel macrolides ABC efflux pump regulated by WhiB7. Future Microbiology. 2019;**14**:47-59. DOI: 10.2217/fmb-2018-0207

[43] Zhang Y, Zhang J, Cui P, Zhang Y, Zhang W. Identification of novel efflux proteins *Rv0191*, *Rv3756c*, *Rv3008*, and *Rv1667c* involved in pyrazinamide resistance in *Mycobacterium tuberculosis*. Antimicrobial Agents and Chemotherapy. 2017;**61**(8):e00940-17. DOI: 10.1128/AAC.00940-17

[44] Birhanu AG, Gomez-Munoz M, Kalayou S, Riaz T, Lutter T, Yimer SA, et al. Proteome profiling of *Mycobacterium tuberculosis* cells exposed to nitrosative stress. ACS Omega. 2022;**7**(4):3470-3482. DOI: 10.1021/acsomega.1c05923

[45] Gupta AK, Katoch VM, Chauhan DS, Sharma R, Singh M, Venkatesan K, et al. Microarray analysis of efflux pump genes in multidrug-resistant *Mycobacterium tuberculosis* during stress induced by common anti-tuberculous drugs. Microbial Drug Resistance. 2010;**16**(1):21-28. DOI: 10.1089/mdr.2009.0054

[46] Malla S, Niraula NP, Liou K, Sohng JK. Self-resistance mechanism in *Streptomyces peucetius*: Overexpression of drrA, drrB and drrC for doxorubicin enhancement. Microbiological Research. 2010;**165**(4):259-267. DOI: 10.1016/j.micres.2009.04.002

[47] Wetzstein N, Diricks M, Anton TB, Andres S, Kuhns M, Kohl TA, et al. Clinical and genomic features of *Mycobacterium avium* complex: A multi-national European study. Genome Medicine. 2024;**16**(1):86. DOI: 10.1186/s13073-024-01359-8

[48] Rindi L. Efflux pump inhibitors against nontuberculous *Mycobacteria*. International Journal of Molecular Sciences. 2020;**21**(12):4191. DOI: 10.3390/ijms21124191

[49] Li G, Zhang J, Guo Q, Wei J, Jiang Y, Zhao X, et al. Study of efflux pump gene expression in rifampicin-monoresistant *Mycobacterium tuberculosis* clinical isolates. Journal of Antibiotics (Tokyo). 2015;**68**(7):431-435. DOI: 10.1038/ja.2015.9

[50] Pang Y, Lu J, Wang Y, Song Y, Wang S, Zhao Y. Study of the rifampin monoresistance mechanism in *Mycobacterium tuberculosis*.

Antimicrobial Agents and Chemotherapy. 2013;**57**(2):893-900. DOI: 10.1128/AAC.01024-12

[51] Balganesh M, Dinesh N, Sharma S, Kuruppath S, Nair AV, Sharma U. Efflux pumps of *Mycobacterium tuberculosis* play a significant role in antituberculosis activity of potential drug candidates. Antimicrobial Agents and Chemotherapy. 2012;**56**(5):2643-2651. DOI: 10.1128/AAC.06003-11

[52] Sharma S, Kumar M, Sharma S, Nargotra A, Koul S, Khan IA. Piperine as an inhibitor of *Rv1258c*, a putative multidrug efflux pump of *Mycobacterium tuberculosis*. The Journal of Antimicrobial Chemotherapy. 2010;**65**(8):1694-1701. DOI: 10.1093/jac/dkq186

[53] Li G, Zhang J, Guo Q, Jiang Y, Wei J, Zhao LL, et al. Efflux pump gene expression in multidrug-resistant *Mycobacterium tuberculosis* clinical isolates. PLoS One. 2015;**10**(2):e119013. DOI: 10.1371/journal.pone.0119013

[54] Li XZ, Zhang L, Nikaido H. Efflux pump-mediated intrinsic drug resistance in *Mycobacterium smegmatis*. Antimicrobial Agents and Chemotherapy. 2004;**48**(7):2415-2423. DOI: 10.1128/AAC.48.7.2415-2423.2004

[55] Li P, Gu Y, Li J, Xie L, Li X, Xie J. *Mycobacterium tuberculosis* major facilitator superfamily transporters. The Journal of Membrane Biology. 2017;**250**(6):573-585. DOI: 10.1007/s00232-017-9982-x

[56] Doran JL, Pang Y, Mdluli KE, Moran AJ, Victor TC, Stokes RW, et al. *Mycobacterium tuberculosis* efpA encodes an efflux protein of the QacA transporter family. Clinical and Diagnostic Laboratory Immunology. 1997;**4**(1):23-32. DOI: 10.1128/cdli.4.1.23-32.1997

[57] Machado D, Lecorche E, Mougari F, Cambau E, Viveiros M. Insights on *Mycobacterium leprae* efflux pumps and their implications in drug resistance and virulence. Frontiers in Microbiology. 2018;**9**:3072. DOI: 10.3389/fmicb.2018.03072

[58] Ramon-Garcia S, Mick V, Dainese E, Martin C, Thompson CJ, De Rossi E, et al. Functional and genetic characterization of the tap efflux pump in *Mycobacterium bovis* BCG. Antimicrobial Agents and Chemotherapy. 2012;**56**(4):2074-2083. DOI: 10.1128/AAC.05946-11

[59] Silva PE, Bigi F, Santangelo MP, Romano MI, Martin C, Cataldi A, et al. Characterization of P55, a multidrug efflux pump in *Mycobacterium bovis* and *Mycobacterium tuberculosis*. Antimicrobial Agents and Chemotherapy. 2001;**45**(3):800-804. DOI: 10.1128/AAC.45.3.800-804.2001

[60] Machado D, Cannalire R, Santos CS, Manfroni G, Tabarrini O, Cecchetti V, et al. Boosting effect of 2-phenylquinoline efflux inhibitors in combination with macrolides against *Mycobacterium smegmatis* and *Mycobacterium avium*. ACS Infectious Diseases. 2015;**1**(12):593-603. DOI: 10.1021/acsinfecdis.5b00052

[61] Takiff HE, Cimino M, Musso MC, Weisbrod T, Martinez R, Delgado MB, et al. Efflux pump of the proton antiporter family confers low-level fluoroquinolone resistance in *Mycobacterium smegmatis*. Proceedings of the National Academy of Sciences of the United States of America. 1996;**93**(1):362-366. DOI: 10.1073/pnas.93.1.362

[62] Mishra MN, Daniels L. Characterization of the *MSMEG_2631* gene (mmp) encoding a multidrug and

toxic compound extrusion (MATE) family protein in *Mycobacterium smegmatis* and exploration of its polyspecific nature using biolog phenotype microarray. Journal of Bacteriology. 2013;**195**(7):1610-1621. DOI: 10.1128/JB.01724-12

[63] Hasan Z, Razzak SA, Kanji A, Shakoor S, Hasan R. Efflux pump gene single-nucleotide variants associated with resistance in *Mycobacterium tuberculosis* isolates with discrepant drug genotypes. Journal of Global Antimicrobial Resistance. 2024;**38**:128-139. DOI: 10.1016/j.jgar.2024.05.006

[64] Shahi F, Khosravi AD, Tabandeh MR, Salmanzadeh S. Investigation of the *Rv3065*, *Rv2942*, *Rv1258c*, *Rv1410c*, and *Rv2459* efflux pump genes expression among multidrug-resistant *Mycobacterium tuberculosis* clinical isolates. Heliyon. 2021;**7**(7):e7566. DOI: 10.1016/j.heliyon.2021.e07566

[65] De Rossi E, Branzoni M, Cantoni R, Milano A, Riccardi G, Ciferri O. Mmr, a *Mycobacterium tuberculosis* gene conferring resistance to small cationic dyes and inhibitors. Journal of Bacteriology. 1998;**180**(22):6068-6071. DOI: 10.1128/JB.180.22.6068-6071.1998

[66] Gutierrez AV, Richard M, Roquet-Baneres F, Viljoen A, Kremer L. The TetR family transcription factor MAB_2299c regulates the expression of two distinct MmpS-MmpL efflux pumps involved in cross-resistance to clofazimine and bedaquiline in *Mycobacterium abscessus*. Antimicrobial Agents and Chemotherapy. 2019;**63**(10):e01000-19. DOI: 10.1128/AAC.01000-19

[67] Gill WP, Harik NS, Whiddon MR, Liao RP, Mittler JE, Sherman DR. A replication clock for *Mycobacterium tuberculosis*. Nature Medicine. 2009;**15**(2):211-214. DOI: 10.1038/nm.1915

[68] Walter ND, Dolganov GM, Garcia BJ, Worodria W, Andama A, Musisi E, et al. Transcriptional adaptation of drug-tolerant *Mycobacterium tuberculosis* during treatment of human tuberculosis. The Journal of Infectious Diseases. 2015;**212**(6):990-998. DOI: 10.1093/infdis/jiv149

[69] Baek SH, Li AH, Sassetti CM. Metabolic regulation of mycobacterial growth and antibiotic sensitivity. PLoS Biology. 2011;**9**(5):e1001065. DOI: 10.1371/journal.pbio.1001065

[70] Serafini A, Tan L, Horswell S, Howell S, Greenwood DJ, Hunt DM, et al. *Mycobacterium tuberculosis* requires glyoxylate shunt and reverse methylcitrate cycle for lactate and pyruvate metabolism. Molecular Microbiology. 2019;**112**(4):1284-1307. DOI: 10.1111/mmi.14362

[71] Pandey AK, Sassetti CM. Mycobacterial persistence requires the utilization of host cholesterol. Proceedings of the National Academy of Sciences of the United States of America. 2008;**105**(11):4376-4380. DOI: 10.1073/pnas.0711159105

[72] Negi A, Sharma R. The significance of persisters in tuberculosis drug discovery: Exploring the potential of targeting the glyoxylate shunt pathway. European Journal of Medicinal Chemistry. 2024;**265**:116058. DOI: 10.1016/j.ejmech.2023.116058

[73] Barry CR, Boshoff HI, Dartois V, Dick T, Ehrt S, Flynn J, et al. The spectrum of latent tuberculosis: Rethinking the biology and intervention strategies. Nature Reviews. Microbiology. 2009;**7**(12):845-855. DOI: 10.1038/nrmicro2236

[74] Connolly LE, Edelstein PH, Ramakrishnan L. Why is long-term therapy required to cure tuberculosis? PLoS Medicine. 2007;**4**(3):e120. DOI: 10.1371/journal.pmed.0040120

[75] Honer ZBK, Russell DG. Mycobacterial persistence: Adaptation to a changing environment. Trends in Microbiology. 2001;**9**(12):597-605. DOI: 10.1016/s0966-842x(01)02238-7

[76] Chakraborty P, Bajeli S, Kaushal D, Radotra BD, Kumar A. Biofilm formation in the lung contributes to virulence and drug tolerance of *Mycobacterium tuberculosis*. Nature Communications. 2021;**12**(1):1606. DOI: 10.1038/s41467-021-21748-6

[77] Assefa M, Girmay G. *Mycobacterium tuberculosis* biofilms: Immune responses, role in TB pathology, and potential treatment. ImmunoTargets and Therapy. 2024;**13**:335-342. DOI: 10.2147/ITT.S455744

[78] Basaraba RJ, Ojha AK. Mycobacterial biofilms: Revisiting tuberculosis bacilli in ExtraCellular necrotizing lesions. Microbiology Spectrum. 2012;**5**(3):10.1128/microbiolspec.TBTB2-0024-2016

[79] Johansen MD, Herrmann JL, Kremer L. Non-tuberculous mycobacteria and the rise of *Mycobacterium abscessus*. Nature Reviews. Microbiology. 2020;**18**(7):392-407. DOI: 10.1038/s41579-020-0331-1

[80] Teng R, Dick T. Isoniazid resistance of exponentially growing *Mycobacterium smegmatis* biofilm culture. FEMS Microbiology Letters. 2003;**227**(2):171-174. DOI: 10.1016/S0378-1097(03)00584-6

[81] Yamazaki Y, Danelishvili L, Wu M, Hidaka E, Katsuyama T, Stang B, et al. The ability to form biofilm influences *Mycobacterium avium* invasion and translocation of bronchial epithelial cells. Cellular Microbiology. 2006;**8**(5):806-814. DOI: 10.1111/j.1462-5822.2005.00667.x

[82] Marsollier L, Aubry J, Coutanceau E, Andre JP, Small PL, Milon G, et al. Colonization of the salivary glands of Naucoris cimicoides by *Mycobacterium ulcerans* requires host plasmatocytes and a macrolide toxin, mycolactone. Cellular Microbiology. 2005;**7**(7):935-943. DOI: 10.1111/j.1462-5822.2005.00521.x

[83] Bosio S, Leekha S, Gamb SI, Wright AJ, Terrell CL, Miller DV. *Mycobacterium fortuitum* prosthetic valve endocarditis: A case for the pathogenetic role of biofilms. Cardiovascular Pathology. 2012;**21**(4):361-364. DOI: 10.1016/j.carpath.2011.11.001

[84] Abraham EP, Chain E, Fletcher CM, Florey HW, Gardner AD, Heatley NG, et al. Further observations on penicillin. 1941. European Journal of Clinical Pharmacology. 1992;**42**(1):3-9

[85] Chambers HF, Moreau D, Yajko D, Miick C, Wagner C, Hackbarth C, et al. Can penicillins and other beta-lactam antibiotics be used to treat tuberculosis? Antimicrobial Agents and Chemotherapy. 1995;**39**(12):2620-2624. DOI: 10.1128/AAC.39.12.2620

[86] Wang F, Cassidy C, Sacchettini JC. Crystal structure and activity studies of the *Mycobacterium tuberculosis* beta-lactamase reveal its critical role in resistance to beta-lactam antibiotics. Antimicrobial Agents and Chemotherapy. 2006;**50**(8):2762-2771. DOI: 10.1128/AAC.00320-06

[87] Hugonnet JE, Blanchard JS. Irreversible inhibition of the *Mycobacterium tuberculosis*

beta-lactamase by clavulanate. Biochemistry-US. 2007;**46**(43):11998-12004. DOI: 10.1021/bi701506h

[88] Zaunbrecher MA, Sikes RJ, Metchock B, Shinnick TM, Posey JE. Overexpression of the chromosomally encoded aminoglycoside acetyltransferase *eis* confers kanamycin resistance in *Mycobacterium tuberculosis*. Proceedings of the National Academy of Sciences of the United States of America. 2009;**106**(47):20004-20009. DOI: 10.1073/pnas.0907925106

[89] Houghton JL, Green KD, Pricer RE, Mayhoub AS, Garneau-Tsodikova S. Unexpected N-acetylation of capreomycin by mycobacterial Eis enzymes. The Journal of Antimicrobial Chemotherapy. 2013;**68**(4):800-805. DOI: 10.1093/jac/dks497

[90] Nessar R, Cambau E, Reyrat JM, Murray A, Gicquel B. *Mycobacterium abscessus*: A new antibiotic nightmare. The Journal of Antimicrobial Chemotherapy. 2012;**67**(4):810-818. DOI: 10.1093/jac/dkr578

[91] Rominski A, Roditscheff A, Selchow P, Bottger EC, Sander P. Intrinsic rifamycin resistance of *Mycobacterium abscessus* is mediated by ADP-ribosyltransferase MAB_0591. The Journal of Antimicrobial Chemotherapy. 2017;**72**(2):376-384. DOI: 10.1093/jac/dkw466

[92] Quan S, Venter H, Dabbs ER. Ribosylative inactivation of rifampin by *Mycobacterium smegmatis* is a principal contributor to its low susceptibility to this antibiotic. Antimicrobial Agents and Chemotherapy. 1997;**41**(11):2456-2460. DOI: 10.1128/AAC.41.11.2456

[93] Hetherington SV, Watson AS, Patrick CC. Sequence and analysis of the *rpoB* gene of *Mycobacterium smegmatis*. Antimicrobial Agents and Chemotherapy. 1995;**39**(9):2164-2166. DOI: 10.1128/AAC.39.9.2164

[94] Quan S, Imai T, Mikami Y, Yazawa K, Dabbs ER, Morisaki N, et al. ADP-ribosylation as an intermediate step in inactivation of rifampin by a mycobacterial gene. Antimicrobial Agents and Chemotherapy. 1999;**43**(1):181-184. DOI: 10.1128/AAC.43.1.181

[95] Warrier T, Kapilashrami K, Argyrou A, Ioerger TR, Little D, Murphy KC, et al. N-methylation of a bactericidal compound as a resistance mechanism in *Mycobacterium tuberculosis*. Proceedings of the National Academy of Sciences of the United States of America. 2016;**113**(31):E4523-E4530. DOI: 10.1073/pnas.1606590113

[96] Buriankova K, Doucet-Populaire F, Dorson O, Gondran A, Ghnassia JC, Weiser J, et al. Molecular basis of intrinsic macrolide resistance in the *Mycobacterium tuberculosis* complex. Antimicrobial Agents and Chemotherapy. 2004;**48**(1):143-150. DOI: 10.1128/AAC.48.1.143-150.2004

[97] Madsen CT, Jakobsen L, Buriankova K, Doucet-Populaire F, Pernodet JL, Douthwaite S. Methyltransferase Erm(37) slips on rRNA to confer atypical resistance in *Mycobacterium tuberculosis*. The Journal of Biological Chemistry. 2005;**280**(47):38942-38947. DOI: 10.1074/jbc.M505727200

[98] Madsen CT, Jakobsen L, Douthwaite S. *Mycobacterium smegmatis* Erm(38) is a reluctant dimethyltransferase. Antimicrobial Agents and Chemotherapy. 2005;**49**(9):3803-3809. DOI: 10.1128/AAC.49.9.3803-3809.2005

[99] Nash KA, Zhang Y, Brown-Elliott BA, Wallace RJ. Molecular basis of intrinsic macrolide resistance in clinical isolates of *Mycobacterium fortuitum*. The Journal of Antimicrobial Chemotherapy. 2005;**55**(2):170-177. DOI: 10.1093/jac/dkh523

[100] Nash KA, Brown-Elliott BA, Wallace RJ. A novel gene, *erm(41)*, confers inducible macrolide resistance to clinical isolates of *Mycobacterium abscessus* but is absent from *Mycobacterium chelonae*. Antimicrobial Agents and Chemotherapy. 2009;**53**(4):1367-1376. DOI: 10.1128/AAC.01275-08

[101] Hu Y, Morichaud Z, Chen S, Leonetti JP, Brodolin K. *Mycobacterium tuberculosis* RbpA protein is a new type of transcriptional activator that stabilizes the sigma A-containing RNA polymerase holoenzyme. Nucleic Acids Research. 2012;**40**(14):6547-6557. DOI: 10.1093/nar/gks346

[102] Sreevatsan S, Stockbauer KE, Pan X, Kreiswirth BN, Moghazeh SL, Jacobs WJ, et al. Ethambutol resistance in *Mycobacterium tuberculosis*: Critical role of *embB* mutations. Antimicrobial Agents and Chemotherapy. 1997;**41**(8):1677-1681. DOI: 10.1128/AAC.41.8.1677

[103] Hegde SS, Vetting MW, Roderick SL, Mitchenall LA, Maxwell A, Takiff HE, et al. A fluoroquinolone resistance protein from *Mycobacterium tuberculosis* that mimics DNA. Science. 2005;**308**(5727):1480-1483. DOI: 10.1126/Science.1110699

[104] Feng L, Mundy J, Stevenson C, Mitchenall LA, Lawson DM, Mi K, et al. The pentapeptide-repeat protein, MfpA, interacts with mycobacterial DNA gyrase as a DNA T-segment mimic. Proceedings of the National Academy of Sciences of the United States of America. 2021;**118**(11):e2016705118. DOI: 10.1073/pnas.2016705118

[105] Gao S, Wu F, Gurcha SS, Batt SM, Besra GS, Rao Z, et al. Structural analysis of phosphoribosyltransferase-mediated cell wall precursor synthesis in *Mycobacterium tuberculosis*. Nature Microbiology. 2024;**9**(4):976-987. DOI: 10.1038/s41564-024-01643-8

[106] Mikusova K, Slayden RA, Besra GS, Brennan PJ. Biogenesis of the mycobacterial cell wall and the site of action of ethambutol. Antimicrobial Agents and Chemotherapy. 1995;**39**(11):2484-2489. DOI: 10.1128/AAC.39.11.2484

[107] Hong W, Chen L, Xie J. Molecular basis underlying *Mycobacterium tuberculosis* D-cycloserine resistance. Is there a role for ubiquinone and menaquinone metabolic pathways? Expert Opinion on Therapeutic Targets. 2014;**18**(6):691-701. DOI: 10.1517/14728222.2014.902937

[108] Prosser GA, de Carvalho LP. Kinetic mechanism and inhibition of *Mycobacterium tuberculosis* D-alanine: D-alanine ligase by the antibiotic D-cycloserine. The FEBS Journal. 2013;**280**(4):1150-1166. DOI: 10.1111/febs.12108

[109] Desjardins CA, Cohen KA, Munsamy V, Abeel T, Maharaj K, Walker BJ, et al. Genomic and functional analyses of *Mycobacterium tuberculosis* strains implicate ald in D-cycloserine resistance. Nature Genetics. 2016;**48**(5):544-551. DOI: 10.1038/ng.3548

[110] Caceres NE, Harris NB, Wellehan JF, Feng Z, Kapur V, Barletta RG. Overexpression of the D-alanine racemase gene confers resistance to D-cycloserine in *Mycobacterium*

smegmatis. Journal of Bacteriology. 1997;**179**(16):5046-5055. DOI: 10.1128/jb.179.16.5046-5055.1997

[111] Feng Z, Barletta RG. Roles of *Mycobacterium smegmatis* D-alanine: D-alanine ligase and D-alanine racemase in the mechanisms of action of and resistance to the peptidoglycan inhibitor D-cycloserine. Antimicrobial Agents and Chemotherapy. 2003;**47**(1):283-291. DOI: 10.1128/AAC.47.1.283-291.2003

[112] Larsen MH, Vilcheze C, Kremer L, Besra GS, Parsons L, Salfinger M, et al. Overexpression of *inhA*, but not *kasA*, confers resistance to isoniazid and ethionamide in *Mycobacterium smegmatis*, *M. Bovis* BCG and *M. tuberculosis*. Molecular Microbiology. 2002;**46**(2):453-466. DOI: 10.1046/j.1365-2958.2002.03162.x

[113] Morlock GP, Metchock B, Sikes D, Crawford JT, Cooksey RC. ethA, inhA, and katG loci of ethionamide-resistant clinical *Mycobacterium tuberculosis* isolates. Antimicrobial Agents and Chemotherapy. 2003;**47**(12):3799-3805. DOI: 10.1128/AAC.47.12.3799-3805.2003

[114] Colangeli R, Helb D, Sridharan S, Sun J, Varma-Basil M, Hazbon MH, et al. The *Mycobacterium tuberculosis* iniA gene is essential for activity of an efflux pump that confers drug tolerance to both isoniazid and ethambutol. Molecular Microbiology. 2005;**55**(6):1829-1840. DOI: 10.1111/j.1365-2958.2005.04510.x

[115] Hartkoorn RC, Uplekar S, Cole ST. Cross-resistance between clofazimine and bedaquiline through upregulation of MmpL5 in *Mycobacterium tuberculosis*. Antimicrobial Agents and Chemotherapy. 2014;**58**(5):2979-2981. DOI: 10.1128/AAC.00037-14

[116] Bloemberg GV, Keller PM, Stucki D, Trauner A, Borrell S, Latshang T, et al. Acquired resistance to bedaquiline and delamanid in therapy for tuberculosis. The New England Journal of Medicine. 2015;**373**(20):1986-1988. DOI: 10.1056/NEJMc1505196

[117] Halloum I, Viljoen A, Khanna V, Craig D, Bouchier C, Brosch R, et al. Resistance to thiacetazone derivatives active against *Mycobacterium abscessus* involves mutations in the MmpL5 transcriptional repressor MAB_4384. Antimicrobial Agents and Chemotherapy. 2017;**61**(4):e02509-16. DOI: 10.1128/AAC.02509-16

[118] Richard M, Gutierrez AV, Viljoen AJ, Ghigo E, Blaise M, Kremer L. Mechanistic and structural insights into the unique TetR-dependent regulation of a drug efflux pump in *Mycobacterium abscessus*. Frontiers in Microbiology. 2018;**9**:649. DOI: 10.3389/fmicb.2018.00649

[119] Telenti A, Imboden P, Marchesi F, Lowrie D, Cole S, Colston MJ, et al. Detection of rifampicin-resistance mutations in *Mycobacterium tuberculosis*. Lancet. 1993;**341**(8846):647-650. DOI: 10.1016/0140-6736(93)90417-f

[120] Campbell EA, Korzheva N, Mustaev A, Murakami K, Nair S, Goldfarb A, et al. Structural mechanism for rifampicin inhibition of bacterial rna polymerase. Cell. 2001;**104**(6):901-912. DOI: 10.1016/s0092-8674(01)00286-0

[121] Rozwarski DA, Grant GA, Barton DH, Jacobs WJ, Sacchettini JC. Modification of the NADH of the isoniazid target (InhA) from *Mycobacterium tuberculosis*. Science. 1998;**279**(5347):98-102. DOI: 10.1126/Science.279.5347.98

[122] Vilcheze C, Wang F, Arai M, Hazbon MH, Colangeli R, Kremer L, et al. Transfer of a point mutation in

Mycobacterium tuberculosis inhA resolves the target of isoniazid. Nature Medicine. 2006;**12**(9):1027-1029. DOI: 10.1038/nm1466

[123] Sun YJ, Luo JT, Wong SY, Lee AS. Analysis of rpsL and rrs mutations in Beijing and non-Beijing streptomycin-resistant *Mycobacterium tuberculosis* isolates from Singapore. Clinical Microbiology and Infection. 2010;**16**(3):287-289. DOI: 10.1111/j.1469-0691.2009.02800.x

[124] Musser JM. Antimicrobial agent resistance in mycobacteria: Molecular genetic insights. Clinical Microbiology Reviews. 1995;**8**(4):496-514. DOI: 10.1128/CMR.8.4.496

[125] Deng L, Mikusova K, Robuck KG, Scherman M, Brennan PJ, McNeil MR. Recognition of multiple effects of ethambutol on metabolism of mycobacterial cell envelope. Antimicrobial Agents and Chemotherapy. 1995;**39**(3):694-701. DOI: 10.1128/AAC.39.3.694

[126] Wolucka BA, McNeil MR, de Hoffmann E, Chojnacki T, Brennan PJ. Recognition of the lipid intermediate for arabinogalactan/arabinomannan biosynthesis and its relation to the mode of action of ethambutol on mycobacteria. The Journal of Biological Chemistry. 1994;**269**(37):23328-23335

[127] Zhao LL, Sun Q, Liu HC, Wu XC, Xiao TY, Zhao XQ, et al. Analysis of embCAB mutations associated with ethambutol resistance in multidrug-resistant *Mycobacterium tuberculosis* isolates from China. Antimicrobial Agents and Chemotherapy. 2015;**59**(4):2045-2050. DOI: 10.1128/AAC.04933-14

[128] Huang WL, Chi TL, Wu MH, Jou R. Performance assessment of the GenoType MTBDRsl test and DNA sequencing for detection of second-line and ethambutol drug resistance among patients infected with multidrug-resistant *Mycobacterium tuberculosis*. Journal of Clinical Microbiology. 2011;**49**(7):2502-2508. DOI: 10.1128/JCM.00197-11

[129] Chen TC, Lu PL, Lin CY, Lin WR, Chen YH. Fluoroquinolones are associated with delayed treatment and resistance in tuberculosis: A systematic review and meta-analysis. International Journal of Infectious Diseases. 2011;**15**(3):e211-e216. DOI: 10.1016/j.ijid.2010.11.008

[130] Lau RW, Ho PL, Kao RY, Yew WW, Lau TC, Cheng VC, et al. Molecular characterization of fluoroquinolone resistance in *Mycobacterium tuberculosis*: Functional analysis of *gyrA* mutation at position 74. Antimicrobial Agents and Chemotherapy. 2011;**55**(2):608-614. DOI: 10.1128/AAC.00920-10

[131] Malik S, Willby M, Sikes D, Tsodikov OV, Posey JE. New insights into fluoroquinolone resistance in *Mycobacterium tuberculosis*: Functional genetic analysis of *gyrA* and *gyrB* mutations. PLoS One. 2012;**7**(6):e39754. DOI: 10.1371/journal.pone.0039754

[132] Wei W, Zhao Y, Zhang C, Yu M, Wu Z, Xu L, et al. Whole-genome sequencing and transcriptome-characterized *in vitro* evolution of aminoglycoside resistance in *Mycobacterium tuberculosis*. Microbial Genomics. May 2023;**9**(5):mgen001022. DOI: 10.1099/mgen.0.001022

[133] Minuk LM, Brode SK, Mehrabi M, Sharma MK, Stobart M, Soualhine H, et al. Phenotypic amikacin resistance may not indicate poor response to amikacin in *Mycobacterium avium* complex pulmonary disease. Antimicrobial

Agents and Chemotherapy. 2024;**68**(6):e0008424. DOI: 10.1128/aac.00084-24

[134] Cao YJ, Navas MJ, Tortola FM. Analysis of phenotypic and genotypic susceptibility to clarithromycin and amikacin of *Mycobacterium abscessus* complex strains isolated from cystic fibrosis patients. Microorganisms. 2023;**11**(12):2897. DOI: 10.3390/microorganisms11122897

[135] Farhat MR, Freschi L, Calderon R, Ioerger T, Snyder M, Meehan CJ, et al. GWAS for quantitative resistance phenotypes in *Mycobacterium tuberculosis* reveals resistance genes and regulatory regions. Nature Communications. 2019;**10**(1):2128. DOI: 10.1038/s41467-019-10110-6

[136] Johansen SK, Maus CE, Plikaytis BB, Douthwaite S. Capreomycin binds across the ribosomal subunit interface using *tlyA*-encoded 2'-O-methylations in 16S and 23S rRNAs. Molecular Cell. 2006;**23**(2):173-182. DOI: 10.1016/j.molcel.2006.05.044

[137] Swaney SM, Aoki H, Ganoza MC, Shinabarger DL. The oxazolidinone linezolid inhibits initiation of protein synthesis in bacteria. Antimicrobial Agents and Chemotherapy. 1998;**42**(12):3251-3255. DOI: 10.1128/AAC.42.12.3251

[138] Moellering RJ. A novel antimicrobial agent joins the battle against resistant bacteria. Annals of Internal Medicine. 1999;**130**(2):155-157. DOI: 10.7326/0003-4819-130-2-199901190-00012

[139] Xiong L, Kloss P, Douthwaite S, Andersen NM, Swaney S, Shinabarger DL, et al. Oxazolidinone resistance mutations in 23S rRNA of *Escherichia coli* reveal the central region of domain V as the primary site of drug action. Journal of Bacteriology. 2000;**182**(19):5325-5331. DOI: 10.1128/JB.182.19.5325-5331.2000

[140] Meka VG, Pillai SK, Sakoulas G, Wennersten C, Venkataraman L, DeGirolami PC, et al. Linezolid resistance in sequential *Staphylococcus aureus* isolates associated with a T2500A mutation in the 23S rRNA gene and loss of a single copy of rRNA. The Journal of Infectious Diseases. 2004;**190**(2):311-317. DOI: 10.1086/421471

[141] Prystowsky J, Siddiqui F, Chosay J, Shinabarger DL, Millichap J, Peterson LR, et al. Resistance to linezolid: Characterization of mutations in rRNA and comparison of their occurrences in vancomycin-resistant enterococci. Antimicrobial Agents and Chemotherapy. 2001;**45**(7):2154-2156. DOI: 10.1128/AAC.45.7.2154-2156.2001

[142] Beckert P, Hillemann D, Kohl TA, Kalinowski J, Richter E, Niemann S, et al. *rplC* T460C identified as a dominant mutation in linezolid-resistant *Mycobacterium tuberculosis* strains. Antimicrobial Agents and Chemotherapy. 2012;**56**(5):2743-2745. DOI: 10.1128/AAC.06227-11

[143] Gygli SM, Borrell S, Trauner A, Gagneux S. Antimicrobial resistance in *Mycobacterium tuberculosis*: Mechanistic and evolutionary perspectives. FEMS Microbiology Reviews. 2017;**41**(3):354-373. DOI: 10.1093/femsre/fux011

[144] Zhang Y, Heym B, Allen B, Young D, Cole S. The catalase-peroxidase gene and isoniazid resistance of *Mycobacterium tuberculosis*. Nature. 1992;**358**(6387):591-593. DOI: 10.1038/358591a0

[145] Banerjee A, Dubnau E, Quemard A, Balasubramanian V, Um KS, Wilson T, et al. *inhA*, a gene encoding a target for isoniazid and ethionamide in *Mycobacterium tuberculosis*. Science.

1994;**263**(5144):227-230. DOI: 10.1126/Science.8284673

[146] Minato Y, Thiede JM, Kordus SL, McKlveen EJ, Turman BJ, Baughn AD. *Mycobacterium tuberculosis* folate metabolism and the mechanistic basis for para-aminosalicylic acid susceptibility and resistance. Antimicrobial Agents and Chemotherapy. 2015;**59**(9):5097-5106. DOI: 10.1128/AAC.00647-15

[147] DeBarber AE, Mdluli K, Bosman M, Bekker LG, Barry CR. Ethionamide activation and sensitivity in multidrug-resistant *Mycobacterium tuberculosis*. Proceedings of the National Academy of Sciences of the United States of America. 2000;**97**(17):9677-9682. DOI: 10.1073/pnas.97.17.9677

[148] Rodrigues L, Sampaio D, Couto I, Machado D, Kern WV, Amaral L, et al. The role of efflux pumps in macrolide resistance in *Mycobacterium avium* complex. International Journal of Antimicrobial Agents. 2009;**34**(6):529-533. DOI: 10.1016/j.ijantimicag.2009.07.010

[149] Scorpio A, Zhang Y. Mutations in *pncA*, a gene encoding pyrazinamidase/nicotinamidase, cause resistance to the antituberculous drug pyrazinamide in tubercle bacillus. Nature Medicine. 1996;**2**(6):662-667. DOI: 10.1038/nm0696-662

[150] Zhang Y, Shi W, Zhang W, Mitchison D. Mechanisms of pyrazinamide action and resistance. Microbiology Spectrum. 2014;**2**(4):M2-M23. DOI: 10.1128/Microbiolspec.MGM2-0023-2013

[151] Njire M, Tan Y, Mugweru J, Wang C, Guo J, Yew W, et al. Pyrazinamide resistance in *Mycobacterium tuberculosis*: Review and update. Advances in Medical Sciences. 2016;**61**(1):63-71. DOI: 10.1016/j.advms.2015.09.007

[152] Zheng J, Rubin EJ, Bifani P, Mathys V, Lim V, Au M, et al. Para-aminosalicylic acid is a prodrug targeting dihydrofolate reductase in *Mycobacterium tuberculosis*. The Journal of Biological Chemistry. 2013;**288**(32):23447-23456. DOI: 10.1074/jbc.M113.475798

[153] Zhao F, Wang XD, Erber LN, Luo M, Guo AZ, Yang SS, et al. Binding pocket alterations in dihydrofolate synthase confer resistance to Para-aminosalicylic acid in clinical isolates of *Mycobacterium tuberculosis*. Antimicrobial Agents and Chemotherapy. 2014;**58**(3):1479-1487. DOI: 10.1128/AAC.01775-13

[154] Hayashi M, Nishiyama A, Kitamoto R, Tateishi Y, Osada-Oka M, Nishiuchi Y, et al. Adduct formation of delamanid with NAD in *Mycobacteria*. Antimicrobial Agents and Chemotherapy. 2020;**64**(5):e01755-19. DOI: 10.1128/AAC.01755-19

[155] Akbari AA, Nasiri MJ, Pakzad P, Mirsamadi ES. Delamanid and bedaquiline resistance patterns in *Mycobacterium tuberculosis* in Iran: A cross-sectional analysis. New Microbes New Infections. 2024;**60-61**:101437. DOI: 10.1016/j.nmni.2024.101437

[156] Gomez-Gonzalez PJ, Perdigao J, Gomes P, Puyen ZM, Santos-Lazaro D, Napier G, et al. Genetic diversity of candidate loci linked to *Mycobacterium tuberculosis* resistance to bedaquiline, delamanid and pretomanid. Scientific Reports. 2021;**11**(1):19431. DOI: 10.1038/s41598-021-98862-4

[157] Yan MY, Li H, Qu YM, Li SS, Zheng D, Guo XP, et al. CRISPR screening and comparative LC-MS analysis identify genes mediating efficacy

of delamanid and pretomanid against *Mycobacterium tuberculosis*. Advanced Science (Weinh). 2024:e2400176. DOI: 10.1002/advs.202400176

[158] Nyang'Wa BT, Berry C, Kazounis E, Motta I, Parpieva N, Tigay Z, et al. A 24-week, all-oral regimen for rifampin-resistant tuberculosis. The New England Journal of Medicine. 2022;**387**(25):2331-2343. DOI: 10.1056/NEJMoa2117166

[159] McKenna L, Frick M, Angami K, Dubula V, Furin J, Harrington M, et al. The 1/4/6x24 campaign to cure tuberculosis quickly. Nature Medicine. 2023;**29**(1):16-17. DOI: 10.1038/s41591-022-02136-z

[160] Farhat M, Cox H, Ghanem M, Denkinger CM, Rodrigues C, Abd EAM, et al. Drug-resistant tuberculosis: A persistent global health concern. Nature Reviews. Microbiology. 2024;**22**:617-635. DOI: 10.1038/s41579-024-01025-1

[161] World Health Organization. WHO Operational Handbook on Tuberculosis. Module 4: Treatment - Drug-Resistant Tuberculosis Treatment. World Health Organization; 2022. Available from: https://www.who.int/publications/i/item/9789240065116

[162] Dartois VA, Rubin EJ. Anti-tuberculosis treatment strategies and drug development: Challenges and priorities. Nature Reviews. Microbiology. 2022;**20**(11):685-701. DOI: 10.1038/s41579-022-00731-y

[163] Yang L, Hu X, Chai X, Ye Q, Pang J, Li D, et al. Opportunities for overcoming tuberculosis: Emerging targets and their inhibitors. Drug Discovery Today. 2022;**27**(1):326-336. DOI: 10.1016/j.drudis.2021.09.003

[164] Shetye GS, Franzblau SG, Cho S. New tuberculosis drug targets, their inhibitors, and potential therapeutic impact. Translational Research. 2020;**220**:68-97. DOI: 10.1016/j.trsl.2020.03.007

[165] Diacon AH, Barry CR, Carlton A, Chen RY, Davies M, de Jager V, et al. A first-in-class leucyl-tRNA synthetase inhibitor, ganfeborole, for rifampicin-susceptible tuberculosis: A phase 2a open-label, randomized trial. Nature Medicine. 2024;**30**(3):896-904. DOI: 10.1038/s41591-024-02829-7

[166] Brown KL, Wilburn KM, Montague CR, Grigg JC, Sanz O, Perez-Herran E, et al. Cyclic AMP-mediated inhibition of cholesterol catabolism in *Mycobacterium tuberculosis* by the novel drug candidate GSK2556286. Antimicrobial Agents and Chemotherapy. 2023;**67**(1):e129422. DOI: 10.1128/aac.01294-22

[167] Renslo AR. Antibacterial oxazolidinones: Emerging structure-toxicity relationships. Expert Review of Anti-Infective Therapy. 2010;**8**(5):565-574. DOI: 10.1586/eri.10.26

[168] Girase R, Ahmad I, Patel H. Bioisosteric modification of linezolid identified the potential *M. tuberculosis* protein synthesis inhibitors to overcome the myelosuppression and serotonergic toxicity associated with linezolid in the treatment of the multi-drug resistance tuberculosis (MDR-TB). Journal of Biomolecular Structure & Dynamics. 2024;**42**(4):2111-2126. DOI: 10.1080/07391102.2023.2203254

[169] Girase RT, Ahmad I, Oh JM, Kim H, Mathew B, Vagolu SK, et al. Repurposing azoles to resolve serotogenic toxicity associated with linezolid to combat multidrug-resistant tuberculosis. ACS Medicinal Chemistry Letters. 2023;**14**(12):1754-1759. DOI: 10.1021/acsmedchemlett.3c00406

[170] Singh A, Somvanshi P, Grover A. Drug repurposing against arabinosyl transferase (EmbC) of *Mycobacterium tuberculosis*: Essential dynamics and free energy minima based binding mechanics analysis. Gene. 2019;**693**:114-126. DOI: 10.1016/j.gene.2019.01.029

[171] Mazlun MH, Sabran SF, Mohamed M, Abu BM, Abdullah Z. Phenolic compounds as promising drug candidates in tuberculosis therapy. Molecules. 2019;**24**(13):2449. DOI: 10.3390/molecules24132449

[172] Cantrell CL, Franzblau SG, Fischer NH. Antimycobacterial plant terpenoids. Planta Medica. 2001;**67**(8):685-694. DOI: 10.1055/s-2001-18365

[173] Garcia A, Bocanegra-Garcia V, Palma-Nicolas JP, Rivera G. Recent advances in antitubercular natural products. European Journal of Medicinal Chemistry. 2012;**49**:1-23. DOI: 10.1016/j.ejmech.2011.12.029

[174] Copp BR, Pearce AN. Natural product growth inhibitors of *Mycobacterium tuberculosis*. Natural Product Reports. 2007;**24**(2):278-297. DOI: 10.1039/b513520f

[175] Uc-Cachon AH, Borges-Argaez R, Said-Fernandez S, Vargas-Villarreal J, Gonzalez-Salazar F, Mendez-Gonzalez M, et al. Naphthoquinones isolated from diospyros anisandra exhibit potent activity against pan-resistant first-line drugs *Mycobacterium tuberculosis* strains. Pulmonary Pharmacology & Therapeutics. 2014;**27**(1):114-120. DOI: 10.1016/j.pupt.2013.08.001

[176] Lechner D, Gibbons S, Bucar F. Plant phenolic compounds as ethidium bromide efflux inhibitors in *Mycobacterium smegmatis*. The Journal of Antimicrobial Chemotherapy. 2008;**62**(2):345-348. DOI: 10.1093/jac/dkn178

[177] Perez-Gonzalez MZ, Gutierrez-Rebolledo GA, Yepez-Mulia L, Rojas-Tome IS, Luna-Herrera J, Jimenez-Arellanes MA. Antiprotozoal, antimycobacterial, and anti-inflammatory evaluation of *Cnidoscolus chayamansa* (Mc Vaugh) extract and the isolated compounds. Biomedicine & Pharmacotherapy. 2017;**89**:89-97. DOI: 10.1016/j.biopha.2017.02.021

[178] Han J, Liu X, Zhang L, Quinn RJ, Feng Y. Anti-mycobacterial natural products and mechanisms of action. Natural Product Reports. 2022;**39**(1):77-89. DOI: 10.1039/d1np00011j

[179] Dong BY, Xu XY, Li SH, Li S, Zeng XT, Wang YM, et al. Effect of *Scutellaria baicalensis* extract on the growth and biofilm formation of *Mycobacterium abscessus*. Journal of Sichuan University (Natural Science Edition). 2023;**60**(4):169-176. DOI: 19907/j.0490-6756.2023.046003

[180] Arai M, Niikawa H, Kobayashi M. Marine-derived fungal sesterterpenes, ophiobolins, inhibit biofilm formation of *Mycobacterium* species. Journal of Natural Medicines. 2013;**67**(2):271-275. DOI: 10.1007/s11418-012-0676-5

[181] Nobrega FL, Costa AR, Kluskens LD, Azeredo J. Revisiting phage therapy: New applications for old resources. Trends in Microbiology. 2015;**23**(4):185-191. DOI: 10.1016/j.tim.2015.01.006

[182] Hatfull GF. Mycobacteriophages. Microbiology Spectrum. 2018;**6**:5. DOI: 10.1128/Microbiolspec.GPP3-0026-2018

[183] Palucci I, Delogu G. Alternative therapies against *Mycobacterium abscessus*

infections. Clinical Microbiology and Infection. 2024;**30**(6):732-737. DOI: 10.1016/j.cmi.2023.10.001

[184] Dedrick RM, Abad L, Storey N, Kaganovsky AM, Smith BE, Aull HA, et al. The problem of *Mycobacterium abscessus* complex: Multi-drug resistance, bacteriophage susceptibility and potential healthcare transmission. Clinical Microbiology and Infection. 2023;**29**(10):1335-1339. DOI: 10.1016/j.cmi.2023.06.026

[185] Hatfull GF. Mycobacteriophages: From petri dish to patient. PLoS Pathogens. 2022;**18**(7):e1010602. DOI: 10.1371/journal.ppat.1010602

[186] Dedrick RM, Smith BE, Cristinziano M, Freeman KG, Jacobs-Sera D, Belessis Y, et al. Phage therapy of mycobacterium infections: Compassionate use of phages in 20 patients with drug-resistant mycobacterial disease. Clinical Infectious Diseases. 2023;**76**(1):103-112. DOI: 10.1093/cid/ciac453

[187] Nick JA, Dedrick RM, Gray AL, Vladar EK, Smith BE, Freeman KG, et al. Host and pathogen response to bacteriophage engineered against *Mycobacterium abscessus* lung infection. Cell. 2022;**185**(11):1860-1874. DOI: 10.1016/j.Cell.2022.04.024

[188] Dedrick RM, Guerrero-Bustamante CA, Garlena RA, Russell DA, Ford K, Harris K, et al. Engineered bacteriophages for treatment of a patient with a disseminated drug-resistant *Mycobacterium abscessus*. Nature Medicine. 2019;**25**(5):730-733. DOI: 10.1038/s41591-019-0437-z

[189] Zaczek M, Lusiak-Szelachowska M, Jonczyk-Matysiak E, Weber-Dabrowska B, Miedzybrodzki R, Owczarek B, et al. Antibody production in response to staphylococcal MS-1 phage cocktail in patients undergoing phage therapy. Frontiers in Microbiology. 2016;**7**:1681. DOI: 10.3389/fmicb.2016.01681

Chapter 4

Relevance of Efflux Pumps in the Development of Drug Resistance in Mycobacterial Infections

Julieta Luna-Herrera, Axhell Aleid Cornejo-Báez and Karen Delgadillo-Gutiérrez

Abstract

Mycobacteria, including nontuberculous mycobacteria (NTM) and *Mycobacterium tuberculosis* complex (MTB), are global pathogens of major concern due to their intrinsic drug resistance and their capacity to cause a wide range of severe infections. The treatment of mycobacterial infections is particularly challenging because of the multidrug resistance. Efflux pumps are involved in drug resistance by actively expelling antibiotics. A promising strategy to decrease drug resistance is the inhibition of efflux pump activity by efflux pump inhibitors. In this chapter, we will review the current knowledge on efflux pumps and their impact on clinical drug resistance, as well as the potential of efflux pump inhibitors to mitigate resistance. The search for novel compounds as efflux pump inhibitors or the inclusion of existing inhibitors in the current drug therapy for mycobacterial infections has become a major goal in the treatment of these diseases.

Keywords: *mycobacteria*, efflux pumps, multidrug resistance, pump inhibitors, efflux resistance mechanism

1. Introduction

There are over 200 distinct species of *Mycobacterium* genus, some of which are economically and clinically important pathogens of humans or animals [1]. Among the human mycobacterial infections, those caused by *M. tuberculosis* (tuberculosis), *M. leprae* (leprosy), and *M. abscessus* (chronic pulmonary infections) pose a public health concern [2]. *Mycobacterial* infections affect 11–14 million people each year globally, and tuberculosis (TB) alone is responsible for an estimated 1.25 million deaths each year. Resistance to rifampicin and isoniazid, the most effective first-line anti-TB drugs, is of greatest concern. TB resistant to rifampicin and isoniazid is defined as Multidrug-Resistant TB (MDR-TB). The estimated annual number of people who developed MDR-TB was 400,000 cases in 2023 [3]. The emergence of antibiotic-resistant strains and rapid spread due to globalization poses a serious challenge to global health.

Mycobacteria are a very particular group of bacteria, with a highly hydrophobic cell wall composed of molecules characteristic of the genus *Mycobacterium*: fatty acids known as mycolic acids, waxes such as dimycocerosates, glycolipid compounds such as trehalose dimycolates or glycopeptidolipids, and mannose- and arabinose-based polysaccharides such as lipoarabinomannan that form an external structure to the bacterium similar to a "lipid capsule" called by some authors mycocapsule [4, 5] or as a type of external membrane called "mycomembrane" [6]. The hydrophobic cell wall of mycobacteria represents a key factor contributing to the low susceptibility of this bacterial group to many of the available antibiotics by preventing their penetration into the bacterium and thus exerting their inhibitory effect [7]. Other mechanisms contributing to antibiotic resistance in mycobacteria are the development of genomic mutations that modify the molecular targets on which they act [8]. The development of these mutations generates high levels of drug resistance [9]. In addition, the modification of antibiotics by mycobacteria results in the modified molecule not binding to its target (**Figure 1**) [7].

Another mechanism in drug resistance is the expression of efflux pumps, whose activity decreases the intracellular concentration of drugs by expelling antibiotics. Also, these pumps remove other substances harmful to bacteria such as metals, disinfectants, or dyes (**Figure 2**) [10]. In this chapter, we will review the impact of efflux pumps expressed by mycobacteria in developing multidrug resistance, which largely contributed to the resurgence of this disease and its declaration as a global health emergency by the World Health Organization [3].

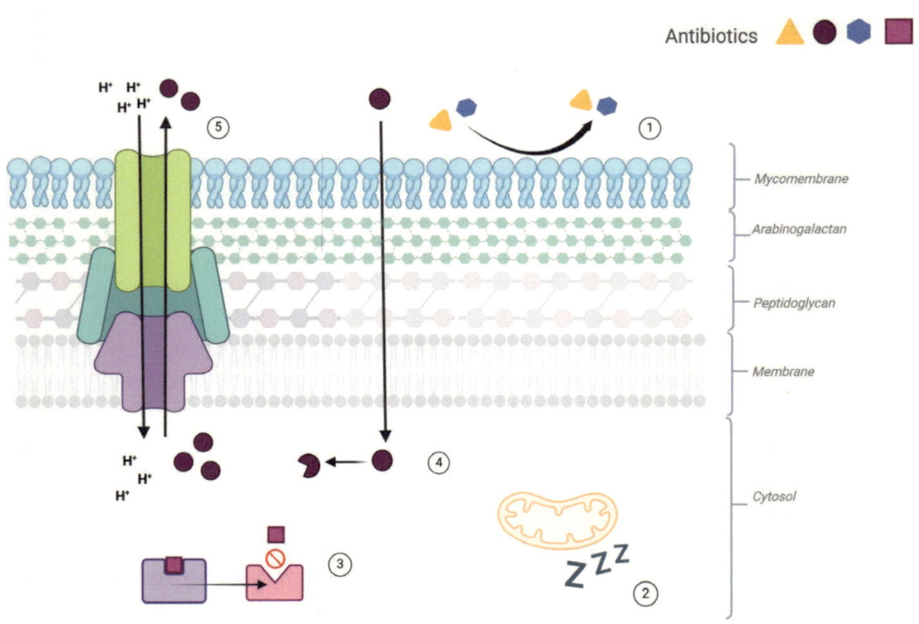

Figure 1.
Drug-resistant mechanisms in mycobacteria. (1) The hydrophobic cell wall of mycobacteria "mycomembrane"; (2) Dormancy; (3) Target modification; (4) Modification of antibiotics; (5) Expression of efflux pumps.

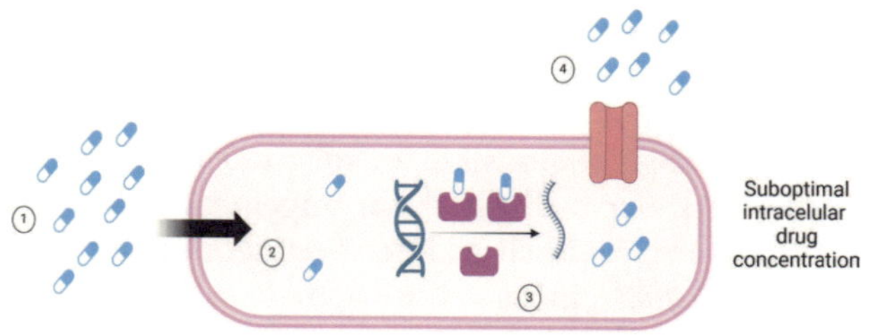

Figure 2.
Effect of efflux pumps on intracellular antibiotic concentration. (1) Antibiotics enter the cell by different mechanisms (diffusion, porin-type channels, active transport, diffusion facilitated by specific carriers, self-promotion of the uptake). (2) Antibiotics accumulate intracellularly. (3) Antibiotics exert their inhibitory effect by binding to their molecular target. (4) Antibiotic expulsion by efflux pumps decreases intracellular drug concentration.

2. Efflux pumps in tuberculous and nontuberculous mycobacteria

Mycobacteria can enter a physiological state in which they develop different mechanisms to tolerate and persist under stress conditions; one of these mechanisms is the expression of efflux pumps. Efflux pumps are a system of proteins anchored in the cell membrane of microorganisms responsible for secreting toxins or metabolites formed by bacteria, as well as effluxing toxic compounds causing bacterial stress, such as antibiotics or dyes [11, 12]. In addition, they directly influence pathogenicity, virulence, biofilm production, and quorum sensing [13, 14]. Efflux pumps conferring resistance to one or more antibiotics have been described in mycobacteria; in fact, the genome of *M. tuberculosis* H37Rv has abundant open reading frames encoding putative efflux proteins [15]. Numerous membrane transporters have been characterized in mycobacteria, including five distinct superfamilies of transporters: ATP-binding cassette (ABC), major facilitator superfamily (MFS), small multidrug resistance (SMR) family, resistance nodulation cleavage (RND), and multidrug and toxic compound extrusion (MATE). Another family of efflux pumps is the proteobacterial antimicrobial compound efflux (PACE), so far not described in mycobacteria [16, 17]. Transporters belonging to the ABC and PACE families utilize energy derived from ATP hydrolysis to drive the efflux of drugs. On the other hand, MFS, SMR, RND, and MATE-type transporters require an energized membrane and proton motive force. Efflux pumps act as uniporters, symporters, and antiporters of protons, metabolites, and drugs [18]. PACE pumps have primarily been identified in gram-negative bacteria, especially proteobacteria, and are involved in the expulsion of antimicrobial compounds [19]. In mycobacteria, the efflux systems characterized so far mainly belong to the ABC, MFS, RND, SMR, and MATE superfamilies. For example, in *M. tuberculosis*, efflux pumps such as Rv1258c (Tap), Rv1410c (P55), and Rv2936 (MmpL7) have been identified, which contribute to multidrug resistance [20].

2.1 ATP-binding cassette (ABC) transporters

ATP-binding cassette transporters are multicomponent primary active transporters of small molecules and macromolecules in response to ATP hydrolysis. *M. tuberculosis* complex species and pathogenic group strains have between 160 and 200 proteins dedicated to ATP-dependent transport systems. In M. *tuberculosis*, 2.5% of the genome is encoded for ABC transporter components. Structurally, ABC transporters consist of two hydrophobic transmembrane domains (TMDs), forming the pore through which the substrate moves, and two cytoplasmic nucleotide-binding domains (NBDs), which provide the energy required for substrate translocation by ATP hydrolysis. In addition, they have a third component, a periplasmic substrate-binding protein (SBP), which is responsible for substrate uptake and delivery to the pores formed by TMDs [21]. According to the arrangement and architecture of the TMDs, the ABC transporters are classified into seven families: three importers and four exporters. In M. *tuberculosis*, most of the importer systems belong to group I, which transports sugars, amino acids, peptides, and anions. Group II comprises systems related to the import of iron, and group III includes a single cobalt transporter. On the other hand, ABC export systems in *M. tuberculosis* are divided into groups IV, V, and VII [21–23]. Genomic sequence analyses of *M. tuberculosis* identified at least 12 putative ABC transporters: Rv0194, Rv1218c-Rv1217c, drrA-drrB-drrC, Rv1273c-Rv1272c, Rv2688c-Rv2687c-Rv2686c, Rv1348-Rv1349, Rv1456c-Rv1457c-Rv1458c, Rv1473, Rv1667c-Rv1668c, Rv1686c-Rv1687c, Rv1819, and Rv2477 [20]. The drr operon plays an essential role in the virulence of *M. tuberculosis*, whose function is to export dimycocerosate (DIM), an antigenic lipid, to the cell surface [24].

2.2 Major facilitator superfamily (MFS) transporters

The MFS family, also known as the uniporter-symporter-antiporter family, constitutes the largest group of single polypeptide secondary membrane transporters capable of transporting only small solutes in response to chemiosmotic ionic gradients [25]. Members of the MFS transport sugars, polyols, drugs, neurotransmitters, amino acids, peptides, and inorganic anions; most are substrate-specific. However, six families contain multispecific MDR transporters [26]. MFS MDR transporters are widespread among microbial genomes and act as single-component pumps capable of transporting small solutes across the inner membrane [27]. Based on sequence analysis, at least 16 putative MSF efflux pump genes have been identified in *M. tuberculosis*, including Rv0037c, Rv0191, Rv0783c, Rv0849, Rv1250, Rv1258c, Rv1410c, Rv163, Rv1877, Rv2333c, Rv2456c, Rv2459, Rv2846c (efpA), Rv28994, Rv3239c, and Rv3728 [24]. The putative MFS family protein Rv1877 in *M. tuberculosis* is an efflux pump for multiple drugs, such as fluoroquinolones, and contributes to biofilm formation [28].

2.3 Small multidrug resistance (SMR) family

The SMR family of proteins is one of the five protein families that comprise the drug/metabolite transporter superfamily. They are integral inner membrane proteins with a length between 100 and 140 amino acids (~12 kDa). These proteins consist of four transmembrane α-helices with short hydrophilic loops that make them very hydrophobic, a feature that allows their solubilization in organic solvents [29, 30]. Four functional subtypes of SMRs have been identified to transport the small, charged metabolite guanidinium, bulky hydrophobic drugs and antiseptics, polyamines, and glycolipids across the lipid membrane [31]. In addition, they confer resistance to various quaternary ammonium compounds [29].

2.4 Resistance nodulation division (RND) transporters

RND family transporters are the major drug efflux pumps in gram-negative bacteria; however, they are also widely distributed in mycobacteria [32]. Mycobacterial RND family transporters are termed Mycobacterial membrane proteins (Mmp) and possess operons encoding large (MmpL) and small (MmpS) units [33]. Most members of the MmpL family consist of 11–12 transmembrane domains (TMD) and two periplasmic loop domains (>100 kDa). MmpL transporters are classified into two groups based on structural motifs. Group I comprises MmpL1, 2, 4, 5, 5, 6, 7, 8, 9, 10, and 12 and has a distinguishable predicted docking domain in the periplasmic loop region. Group II comprises MmpL3, 11, and the fusion protein MmpL13a/b [34]. Among the wide range of putative MmpL substrates are the various lipids and mycolic acids in the single mycobacterial envelope, some released from the mycobacterial envelope into the phagosomes of infected macrophages [35]. The primary function of MmpLs is to translocate envelope lipids and virulence-associated complex siderophores across the plasma membrane into the periplasmic space [36, 37]. However, one of the MmpL proteins involved in antibiotic efflux is MmpL7, associated with isoniazid efflux in *M. smegmatis* [38]. **Table 1** describes the MmpL proteins of *M. tuberculosis* and their main functions.

2.5 Multidrug and toxic compound extrusion (MATE) transporters

MATE transporters use H+ or Na + gradients across the membrane to drive substrate export [47] MATE transporters are subclassified by their amino acid sequence similarity into NorM, DinF (DNA damage-inducible F protein), and eukaryotic subfamilies. Many MATE transporters are unable to export negatively charged compounds, but bacterial and human MATE transporters can export various antibiotics, anticancer, and antidiabetic drugs, becoming promising therapeutic targets to address multidrug resistance in pathogens, as well as to control drug-drug interactions in humans [48]. MATE transporters function as multidrug efflux pumps by conferring resistance to structurally diverse antibiotics and DNA-damaging chemicals [49].

2.6 Proteobacterial antimicrobial compound efflux (PACE) transporters

Efflux pumps of the PACE (Proteobacterial Antimicrobial Compound Efflux) family represent a relatively recent class of efflux transporters primarily identified

Mycobacterial MmpL	Role in *M. tuberculosis*	Reference
MmpL2	Unknown substrate.	[39]
MmpL3 (Rv0206c)	Transport of trehalose monomycolate (TMM).	[40]
MmpL4	Export of mycobacterial siderophores.	[41]
MmpL5	Export of mycobacterial siderophores.	[41]
MmpL7 (Rv2442)	Contribution to drug efflux.	[42]
MmpL8 (Rv3823c)	Transport of polyketide phthiocerol dimycocerosate (PDIM). Contribution to drug efflux.	[43]
MmpL9 (Rv2339)	Transport of cell envelope sulfolipid-1.	[44]
MmpL10 (Rv1183)	Involvement in inhibition of phagosomal maturation.	[45]
MmpL11 (Rv0202c)	Translocation of diacyltrehalose (DAT) across the plasma membrane, where it is acylated to produce penta-acyltrehalose.	[46]

Table 1.
Main functions in M. tuberculosis *metabolism of MmpL transporters.*

in gram-negative bacteria, particularly among proteobacteria, though they have also been found in some Actinobacteria and a limited number of other bacterial species [19]. These pumps play a critical role in antimicrobial resistance by expelling a range of toxic compounds, including disinfectants like chlorhexidine and certain antibiotics, using the proton motive force as an energy source [50]. Some natural polyamines, such as cadaverine, putrescine, spermidine, and spermine, exhibit structural similarities to chlorhexidine. Consequently, short-chain diamines serve as common substrates for the PACE family of transport proteins, further underscoring their significance as an emerging class of efflux pumps [51]. PACE transporters consist of proteins of ~150 amino acid residues with four transmembrane helices [52]. While they are considered to have evolved as a defense mechanism against environmental toxins, their presence or functionality has not yet been demonstrated in mycobacteria, highlighting the need for further exploration of their potential role in this genus. This absence underscores the uniqueness of efflux systems in mycobacteria and their distinct strategies for antimicrobial resistance. In short, **Table 2** shows the families of mycobacterial efflux pumps, the genes that encode them, and the antibiotics they expel.

In a study by Narang *et al.*, the role of four efflux pumps (MmpL2, MmpL5, Rv0194, and Rv1250) in rifampicin (RIF) resistance in *M. tuberculosis* was investigated. The researchers analyzed the expression of these pumps in 16 RIF-resistant and 11 RIF-susceptible clinical strains after exposure to RIF. They found that Rv0194 and MmpL5 were expressed at higher levels in RIF-resistant isolates compared to susceptible ones. However, no direct association between these efflux pumps and RIF resistance was identified, suggesting that the overexpression of Rv0194 and MmpL5 in resistance isolates warrants further investigation [70]. **Table 2** shows the families of mycobacterial efflux pumps, the gene that encodes them, and which antibiotic they expel.

Efflux pump family	Efflux pump gene	*Mycobacterium*	Antibiotic to which it provides resistance	Reference
ABC	Rv0194	*M. tuberculosis*	AMP, VCM, NVC, ETM, CLF, STR, TCL	[53]
		M. smegmatis		
		M. bovis		
	Rv0450	*M. tuberculosis*	INH y RIF	[54]
	Rv1217c-Rv1218c	*M. tuberculosis*	INH, RIF	[54]
	Rv1272c-Rv1273c	*M. tuberculosis*	INH, RIF, ETB, FLQ, CFC, AMK, GEN	[55]
	Rv1457	*M. tuberculosis*	RIF y ETB	[56]
	Rv1458	*M. tuberculosis*	INH y RIF	[54]
	bacA (Rv1819c)	*M. tuberculosis*	INH, RIF, STR	[56, 57]
	Rv2477	*M. tuberculosis*	OXO	[57]
	Rv2688	*M. tuberculosis*	FLQ	[54]
	drrA	*M. tuberculosis*	RIF	[58]
	drrB (Rv2937)	*M. tuberculosis*	INH, RIF	[54, 58]
	drrC (Rv2938)	*M. tuberculosis*	STR	[57]

Efflux pump family	Efflux pump gene	*Mycobacterium*	Antibiotic to which it provides resistance	Reference
MFS	Rv0191	*M. tuberculosis*	CLF	[59]
	Rv0842	*M. tuberculosis*	RIF y ETB	[56]
	P55 (Rv1410)	*M. tuberculosis*	TCL, STR, GTM	[15]
		M. abscessuss	CLR	[60]
	Rv1634	*M. tuberculosis*	INH, RIF, ETB	[56]
	Rv1877	*M. tuberculosis*	FLQ	[28]
	EfpA	*M. tuberculosis*	INH, RIF, CIP, OXO y AMK	[61, 62]
		M. smegmatis	RIF, CIP	[61]
		M. abscessus	CLR	[60]
	tap (Rv 1258c)	*M. tuberculosis*	INH, RIF, TCL y CFZ	[63]
		M. bovis	ETM	[64]
		M. smegmatis	INH, RIF, ETB, PZA	[64]
		M. abscessus	CLR	[60]
	LfrA	*M. smegmatis*	FLQ	[65]
	Tet (V)	*M. smegmatis*	TCL	[66]
	jefA (Rv2459)	*M. tuberculosis*	INH, ETB, RIF,	[67]
	Rv3728	*M. tuberculosis*	INH y RIF	[57]
	Rv3827	*M. tuberculosis*	INH y RIF	[54]
	Rv2333c (stp)	*M. tuberculosis*	RIF, TCL, EPMC	[54, 58, 68]
RND	mmpS-MmpL	*M. abscessus*	CFZ, BDQ	[69]
	mmpL2 (Rv0507)	*M. tuberculosis*	INH y RIF	[54]
	mmpL5 (Rv0676c)	*M. tuberculosis*	INH y RIF	[54]
	mmpL8 (Rv3823)	*M. tuberculosis*	RIF, ETB	[56]
SMR	mmr RV305	*M. tuberculosis*	INH y ETB	[57]
MATE	dinF (mmp)	All mycobacteria *(except M. leprae)*	FLMC, BLMC, CPMC, AMK, SFM	[49]

AMP = Ampicillin; AMK = Amikacin; GEN = Gentamicin; VCM = Vancomycin; NVC = Novobiocin; ERM = Erythromycin; CLF = Chloramphenicol; INH = Isoniazid; RIF = Rifampicin; ETB = Ethambutol; PZA = Pyrazinamide; FLQ = Fluoroquinolones; CIP = Ciprofloxacin; OXO = Oxofloxacin; STR = Streptomycin; TCL = Tetracycline; CFZ = Clofazimine; BDQ = Bedaquiline; EPMC = Spectinomycin; FLMC = Phleomycin; BLMC = Bleomycin; CPMC = Capreomycin; SFM = Sulfamides.

Table 2.
Putative transporters in the membrane of Mycobacteria *and the antibiotics they expel.*

3. Efflux pump inhibitors

One of the major causes of multidrug resistance in bacteria is through efflux pumps. Nevertheless, a promising strategy to decrease drug resistance and multidrug resistance in mycobacterial infections is the inhibition of efflux pump activity by efflux pump inhibitors [71, 72]. Efflux pump inhibitors are compounds from various natural and synthetic sources that efficiently block efflux pumps [73]. Different efflux pump inhibitors exhibit different modes of action that can be either broad or specific to one class of efflux pump (**Table 3**) [74].

Several mechanisms of efflux pump inhibition have been reported, such as inhibition or down-regulation of efflux pump expression, blockage of the assembly of protein components of efflux pumps, inhibition of the pump's energy source, inhibition of phosphorylation steps, application of antibodies against pump proteins or other protein components of efflux pumps, blockage of the efflux pump channel or the outer membrane protein exit channel, application of a small mimic molecule that is recognized and effluxes in preference to the antibiotic, application of small efflux pump inhibitory molecules that competitively block the efflux pump drug-binding site and that exert steric hindrance of substrate access to the binding site, as well as application of small efflux pump inhibitory molecules that non-competitively inhibit the essential conformational changes of efflux pumps during the efflux process (**Figure 3**) [75, 76].

Diverse molecules have been described as potential efflux pump inhibitors to enhance the activity of antimicrobials. If the antibiotic is coadministered along with an efflux pump inhibitor, the compound becomes effective again, even in resistant microorganisms. Compounds with inhibitory activity against mycobacterial efflux

Source	Inhibitor type	Representative drugs	Efflux pumps
Plants	Alkaloids	Reserpine	NorA
		Berberine	MexXY-OprM and NorA
		Piperine	NorA, MdeA, and Rv1258c
		Astragalusin, kaempferol, silymarin	NorA
	Flavonoids	Chalcone	NorA and MepA
		Lignocaine	MsrA
	Phenolic metabolites	5′-MHC	NorA
	Fermentation products	EA-371α and EA-371	MexAB-OprM
	Gallic acid	Epigallocatechin gallate	TetK, MexAB-OprM, and CmeABC
Chemical synthesis	Pyranopyridine	MBX2319	AcrAB-TolC
	Peptides	Phe-Arg-β-naphthylamide	MexAB-OprM, MexEF-OprN and MexCD-OprJ
	Phenothiazines	Chlorpromazine	AcrB
	Aryl piperazine derivatives	NMP	AcrAB and AcrEF
	Pyridopyrimidine derivatives	D13-9001	AcrB and MexB

Modified from Zhang et al. [73].

Table 3.
Types of efflux pump inhibitors.

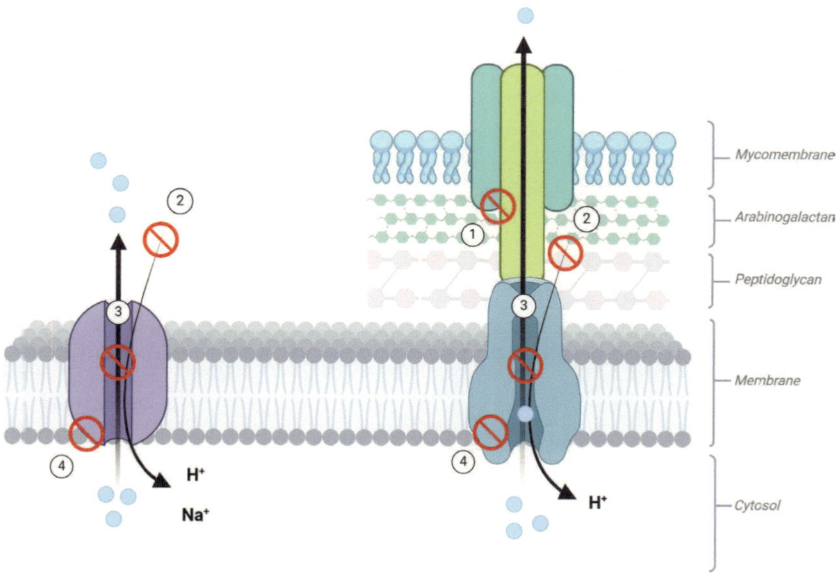

Figure 3.
The major mechanisms of efflux pump inhibitors. (1) Blocking of the assembly of efflux pumps by targeting protein-protein interfaces. (2) Inhibiting the electrochemical gradient by the decrease of the ATP supply or the inhibition of the proton motive force. (3) Blocking the efflux pump channel or outer membrane protein exit channel. (4) Interfering either with the binding site of efflux pump substrates or inhibiting the essential conformational changes during the efflux process.

pumps also show antimicrobial activity; some have antipsychotic properties and are used as antidepressants, anxiolytics, and/or antihypertensives in clinical practice (**Table 4**) [77].

3.1 Calcium channel blockers

Verapamil and phenothiazines inhibit efflux pump activity by reduction of the transmembrane potential. *In vitro* and *in vivo* studies have shown that these compounds inhibit the activity of efflux pumps belonging to the MFS in *Mycobacteria* [74]. For example, the activity of verapamil enhances the efficacy of bedaquiline; it is the first anti multidrug-resistant TB drug approved by the Food and Drug Administration (FDA). However, drug resistance to bedaquiline has already been reported. In general, verapamil exhibited synergistic effects with a series of anti-TB drugs, decreased the Minimum Inhibitory Concentration (MIC) of the drug, reduced drug resistance, and increased drug retention. In addition, studies with animal models found that verapamil enhanced *M. tuberculosis* removal in infected macrophages inhibited the growth and tolerance of intracellular *M. tuberculosis*, reduced the drug dosage, and shortened the duration of therapy [78]. Verapamil has shown clinical potential as an attractive strategy to enhance the activity of drugs [79]. Several studies demonstrated that verapamil strongly inhibits the efflux of ethidium bromide by *M. smegmatis*, *M. avium* complex, and *M. tuberculosis*. Also, verapamil significantly reduced the MIC values for isoniazid among other drugs in *M. tuberculosis* [77]. Phenothiazine and its derivatives (chlorpromazine, piperidine, and thioridazine) are potential inhibitors of K+ transport and Ca^{2+} channels that can reverse the Multidrug-*resistant* (MDR) phenotype in *M. tuberculosis, M. smegmatis,* and *M. avium* complex. Also, these drugs inhibit the proton motive force dependent

Efflux pump inhibitor	Pharmacological use	Physiological mode of action	Microorganisms
Verapamil	Antihypertensive	Calcium channel blocker	*M. smegmatis; M. avium complex; M. tuberculosis complex*
Thioridazine, chlorpromazine	Antipsychotic		*M. smegmatis; M. avium complex; M. tuberculosis complex*
Cis-(Z)-flupentixol (thioxanthene)	Antipsychotic		*M. avium complex*
Bromperidol, haloperidol	Antipsychotic		*M. smegmatis; M. tuberculosis complex; M. avium complex*
Reserpine	Antihypertensive		*M. smegmatis; M. avium complex; M. tuberculosis complex*
Farnesol	Antipsychotic		*M. smegmatis*
Carbonyl cyanide m-chlorophenylhydrazone	Uncoupler of the proton motive force		*M. avium; M. smegmatis; M. fortuitum*
l-phenylalanyl-l-arginyl-β-naphthylamide	Putative efflux-substrate competitor and outer membrane permeabilizer		*M. tuberculosis*
Modified from Viveiros [77].			

Table 4.
The main compounds reported to have inhibitory activity against efflux pumps in Mycobacteria.

MFS pumps by reducing transmembrane potential. Thioridazine and chlorpromazine reduce clarithromycin and isoniazid resistance in *M. tuberculosis* complex [74]. In addition, the efficacy of first-line drugs is enhanced by supplementary treatment of phenothiazines [80].

3.2 Protonophores

Protonophores, which include carbonyl cyanide m-chlorophenylhydrazone (CCCP), 2,4-dinitrophenol (DNP), and valinomycin, are ionophores that act as chemical inhibitors of oxidative phosphorylation, which in turn serves to inhibit the activity of ATP synthase. Also, these compounds inhibit efflux pump activity by reducing the transmembrane potential. *In vitro* and *in vivo* studies have shown that these compounds largely inhibit the activity of efflux pumps belonging to the MFS in *Mycobacteria* [74]. The studies showed that CCCP decreases the MIC of anti-TB drugs (streptomycin, tetracycline, ofloxacin, isoniazid, and ethambutol), reduces resistance to anti-TB drugs (rifampicin, clofazimine, ciprofloxacin, and azoles), and exhibits a synergistic effect with anti-TB drugs. DNP acts similarly to CCCP [78]. Valinomycin is a non-ribosomal peptide from Streptomyces species that transports potassium ions across biological membranes. Initially, it was developed as an antibiotic compound with antibacterial effects against *M. tuberculosis*; later, it showed a wide range of anti-bacterial activity in in vitro studies [81]. Valinomycin is a potassium-specific efflux pump inhibitor with high selectivity for Na + and K+. It has been shown to inhibit the P55 efflux pump, which relies on transmembrane proton and electrochemical gradients as energy sources for the active export of compounds in *M. tuberculosis* [74].

3.3 Plant-derived efflux pump inhibitors

Plants and their extracts can be potent sources of efflux pump inhibitors. These compounds include alkaloids, flavonoids, and essential oils [75, 76]. Plant-derived efflux pump inhibitors are emerging adjuvants with the potential to synergistically improve the potency of some anti-TB drugs [74].

3.3.1 Alkaloids including reserpine, piperine, and berberine

Reserpine is a promising efflux pump inhibitor that targets the RND superfamily, MFS, and membrane protein classes. Also, reserpine influences the resistance level to numerous anti-TB compounds in mycobacteria. Piperine is used commercially as an inhibitor of enzymes important in drug metabolism and the transport of metabolites and xenobiotics. Studies of piperine and piperidine suggest inhibitory action against active bacterial efflux pumps, including those in mycobacteria. Berberine has weak antibacterial activity when acting alone but has a synergistic effect when combined with other compounds [74]. Some studies showed that berberine potentiated the antimycobacterial properties of antibiotics in nontuberculous mycobacteria [82].

3.3.2 Flavonoids

Flavonoids are plant secondary metabolites; more than 8000 flavonoid-like structures have been reported. Chemically, they are 2-phenyl-benzo-γ-pyrones. Flavonoids have been investigated most frequently for efflux pump inhibitor activity on the NorA pump [75]. One study evaluated the antimicrobial and resistance-modifying profiles of various plant-derived flavonoids in model mycobacterial strains: *M. smegmatis, M. aurum*, and *M. bovis* BCG. The results highlight two polymethoxyflavones, skullcapflavone II and nobiletin, with antimycobacterial and antibiotic resistance-modulating activities as valuable adjuvants in antimycobacterial therapies [83]. Some studies have documented the exhibited inhibition of essential oils on the efflux pump activity and the accumulation of antibiotics as their capability to augment membrane permeability, disrupt cell membranes, and decrease ATP synthesis. It seems a good alternative for developing natural efflux pump inhibitors [76]. Efflux pump inhibitors capable of restoring the effectiveness of available antibiotics are urgently needed. Untapped natural products can be a valuable resource for potential efflux pump inhibitors. Additionally, machine learning can help us to screen new efflux pump inhibitors [10].

There are many potential efflux pump inhibitors under study, but none of them has been used clinically for anti-TB therapy. Although bedaquiline and verapamil are approved by the FDA, their application as anti-TB drugs still needs further investigation. The dosage in combined therapy with the existing first-line anti-TB drugs needs to be determined, and the exact combination and drug side effects remain to be clarified. Drugs currently used in clinical therapy for other diseases, such as verapamil, phenothiazines, and reserpine, have a promising future in anti-TB therapy owing to their definite properties regarding safety. However, their side effects could be an issue in future combination therapy. Natural substances of plant origin, such as piperine and berberine, also have great potential as they are part of the diet. Future research should focus on new drugs and regimens of anti-TB therapy with the combined use of multiple drugs [78].

4. Impact of pump expression on drug resistance

As already described, efflux pumps make up a group of transporters that expel multiple substrates, including antibiotics and other aggressors, are not exclusive to a bacterial group or family, and have an ancestral origin that has been conserved throughout the evolution of each microorganism [10]. The sequencing of bacterial genomes of gram-positive and gram-negative bacteria indicates that between 5 and 10% of their genes are involved in cellular transport, with a large proportion of them encoding efflux pumps [84]; among mycobacteria, the proportion is higher, between 6 and 18%, being one of the bacterial genera with the highest numbers of putative genes for this type of transporter [85]. The involvement of efflux pumps in bacterial drug resistance was initially described in the 1990s for *P. aeruginosa*, where the intrinsic resistance to tetracycline, norfloxacin, and chloramphenicol was due to an efflux phenomenon and not to a higher impermeability of the bacterial outer membrane [86]. The importance of efflux pumps in drug resistance is reinforced by a new finding related to resistance to bedaquiline, a recently approved drug for treating multidrug-resistant *M. tuberculosis* (MTB-MDR), as their overexpression is one of the mechanisms responsible for resistance to this drug. Overexpression is due to mutations in the transcriptional repressor of the MmpL5-MmpS5 operon known as Rv0678c, which is an RND-type pump [87]. Some efflux pumps are expressed constitutively, while others are by a stressor stimulus, such as the presence of an antibiotic [88]. The inducible expression of the pumps is a rapid process [9] that allows early protection against stress-causing agents. The regulation of the expression of efflux pumps is a complex phenomenon at the transcriptional and post-transcriptional level. Once in the presence of antibiotics, the sensors of these molecules initiate a complex signaling resulting in changes in the expression of numerous genes for these efflux transporters [88]. On the other hand, the regulation in the expression of pumps is also given by mutations in genes of repressive transcriptional regulators or the promoters, resulting in a sustained overexpression of the genes of some pumps, as already mentioned in the case of resistance to bedaquiline [89]. The activity of efflux pumps goes beyond the phenomenon of antibiotic expulsion, adding a fundamental role as transporters that contribute to bacterial homeostasis [9] since these transporters contribute to the persistence of microorganisms. For example, they allow the efflux of antimicrobial peptides produced during the immune response [90], contribute to the formation of biofilm, favor invasion, and contribute to virulence and colonization, among other activities (**Figure 4**) [9, 90].

The exclusive activation of the efflux systems is not sufficient to generate a state of clinical resistance but a state of low drug resistance [88] or tolerance [91] that, in turn, allows bacteria to persist at the site of infection in the presence of the antibiotic [9]. The expression of efflux systems is considered a preliminary step in developing high levels of resistance, such as those generated when resistance occurs due to mutations in the target genes of antibiotics. The efflux of antibiotics mediated by the pumps can allow the survival and selection of clones with those chromosomal mutations. This case has been described in mycobacteria for the resistance to isoniazid [92], thus acquiring a state of clinical resistance with high levels of Minimum Inhibitory Concentrations (MIC) to the drugs [93]. It has not been established whether the overexpression of the pumps has a direct effect or favors the development of genomic mutations. However, recently an association has been described for *E. coli* between overexpression in the AcrAB-TolC transporter belonging to the

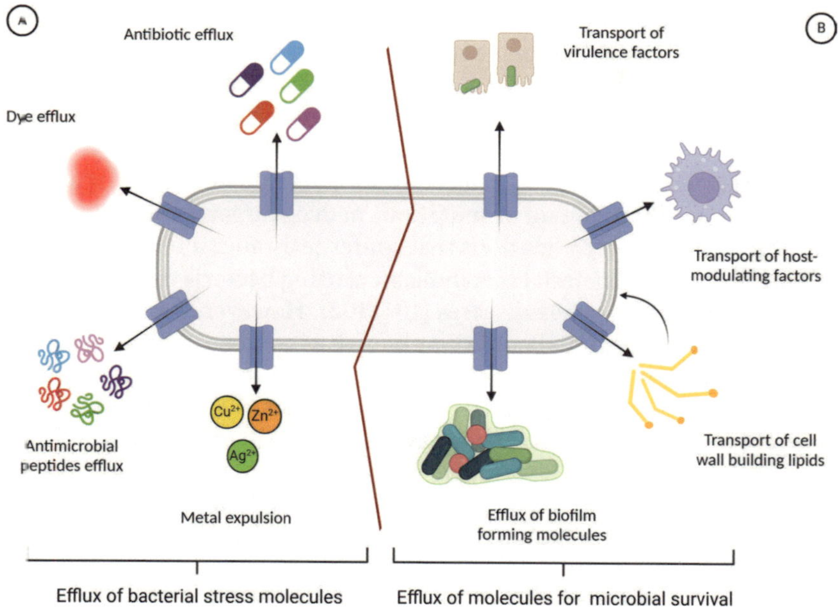

Figure 4.
Biological functions of bacterial efflux pumps. (A) Efflux of bacterial stress molecules due to overexpression of efflux pumps. (B) Efflux of molecules for microbial survival and homeostasis.

RND-type pump family [94] and a general increase in the mutation generation rate [95, 96], a phenomenon attributed to lower expression in the *muts* gene involved in DNA repair [96].

5. The expression of efflux pumps and bacterial fitness

Efflux pumps can be primary and secondary. Primary pumps use energy from the hydrolysis of ATP to expel substrates, while secondary pumps use the proton motive force given by protons and ions for expulsing substrates [10]. The overexpression of both pumps can affect bacterial fitness by increasing energy consumption or decreasing the intracellular pH caused by the excess of protons introduced during the expulsion process [97]. However, this effect does not seem generalized in bacteria, maybe due to the development of metabolic compensation systems that allow microorganisms to survive these circumstances; the recovery process has been called "metabolic rewiring." This phenomenon has been described in *P. aeruginosa*, where the MexEF-OprN operon that encodes an RND-type pump is overexpressed and provokes the overexpression of genes involved in the respiratory chain. It allows *P. aeruginosa* to use nitrates as an electron acceptor under anaerobic conditions, reducing it to nitrogen [98], thus compensating for the possible energetic impact of excess electron influx and its effect on fitness [99]. In mycobacteria, the "metabolic rewiring" describes the metabolic changes made to adapt to different stress situations, including the response to an antibiotic. For example, with isoniazid treatment, mycobacteria alter their lipid metabolism and reduce the production of Reactive Oxygen Species (ROS) levels [91], and with the antibiotics rifampicin and pyrazinamide, the tricarboxylic acid (TCA) metabolic pathway is affected. There are multiple metabolic adaptations with which *M.*

tuberculosis responds to first, second, and third-line antibiotics, including different "metabolic rewiring" among drug-susceptible and drug-resistant clinical isolates of *M. tuberculosis* [100]. However, the metabolic adaptation that mycobacteria carry out to compensate for the overexpression of efflux pumps is not yet fully defined.

It is a well-recognized fact that, in mycobacteria, the phenomenon of acquired resistance due to the development of mutations in drug target genes significantly affects bacterial fitness since mutations that confer resistance alter enzymes or proteins critical for mycobacterial metabolism, causing bacteria to grow more slowly, transmit less, or cause less severe diseases [101, 102]. However, there is evidence that mycobacteria develop additional mutations known as compensatory, which contribute to the recovery of bacterial fitness. Compensatory mutations occur in different genes since they compensate for specific functions affected by the diverse mutations responsible for acquired resistance; they have been described in the case of resistance to isoniazid, rifampicin, streptomycin, fluoroquinolones, and the injectable kanamycin and amikacin, among other antibiotics [103]. Many of the compensatory mutations described so far present a slight-to-medium fitness recovery. However, some mutations allow almost total fitness restoration. These mutations have been found in resistant clinical isolates that have spread in the population; within the latter are compensatory mutations in the *rpoa* and *rpoc* genes that permit the recovery of fitness that has been affected by mutations in the *rpob* gene, responsible for resistance to rifampicin [104–106].

6. Involvement of pump inhibitors in clinical recovery of drug susceptibility

The overexpression of efflux pumps by bacteria subjected to stress caused by antibiotics is a condition that endangers the benefits of antibiotic therapy, so it is essential to develop strategies that interfere with this biological phenomenon. In this sense, efflux pump inhibitors represent a great opportunity not only to interfere with drug expulsion but also to prevent the development of multidrug resistance [9]. Pump inhibitors could also affect bacterial virulence, considering the relevance of these efflux transporters in processes such as biofilm formation [10] or construction of the mycomembrane in mycobacteria [107]. The initial step in the clinical development of drug resistance is a state of antibiotic tolerance promoted partially by efflux pumps that leads to the selection of bacteria with genomic mutations in antibiotic resistance target genes, resulting in clinical resistance (**Figure 5**) [9].

The use of pump inhibitors in clinical therapy is proposed as a mechanism that contributes to antimycobacterial therapy and prevents drug resistance by cutting the chain of events leading to its development. However, very few efflux pump inhibitors have been tested or have been successful in human clinical studies; the reasons for such failures have been toxicity, low *in vivo* efficacy, etc. [108]. Among the pump inhibitors proposed for clinical use in tuberculosis is verapamil, a drug that has been used for the treatment of cardiovascular problems and hypertension [109]. Verapamil is an inhibitor of efflux pumps in *mycobacteria*, favoring the antimycobacterial activity of drugs such as rifampicin at the *in vitro* level [70], at the intracellular level in macrophages [110], and in mouse studies [111]. Its use in humans has been proposed [112] in conjunction with another recently introduced anti-tuberculosis drug, bedaquiline since

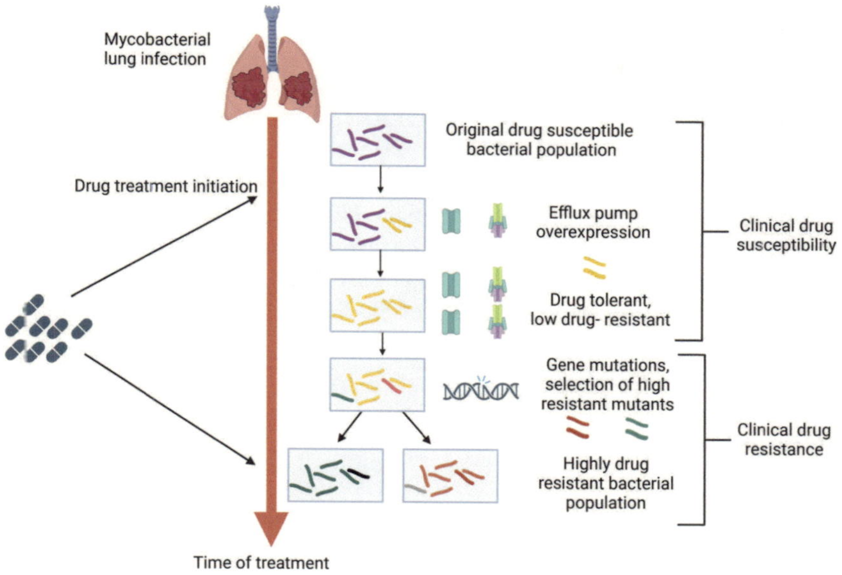

Figure 5.
Impact of efflux pump expression on drug resistance development.

the resistance to this drug is partially due to the expression of an RND-type efflux pump (Mmpl5) [89]. The usefulness of verapamil in the treatment of tuberculosis has not yet been established, but recently the dose of verapamil has been determined to guide its use as adjunct therapy to rifampin in human tuberculosis [112]. Thioridazine is another efflux pump inhibitor that has been suggested as adjunctive therapy for tuberculosis; this is an antipsychotic drug, belonging to the group of phenothiazines [113]. Clinically, thioridazine replaced chlorpromazine, another neuroleptic drug with efflux pump inhibitor properties, widely used in the treatment of schizophrenia and psychosis [114, 115]. The clinical use of thioridazine in combination with linezolid and moxifloxacin was successful in a study performed for compassionate use. In a group of extensively drug-resistant (XDR) tuberculosis patients from Argentina, hematologic disorders and neurotoxicity were observed as side effects, but clinical cure was achieved in 11 out of 17 patients included in the study [116]. In the development of drug resistance, efflux pumps are fundamental; in consequence, the search for pump inhibitors without drug adverse effects is a promising research field.

7. Conclusions

In *mycobacteria*, the overexpression of efflux pumps is a biological phenomenon developed in response to antibiotic therapy. Overexpression of these efflux transporters promotes both a state of tolerance to antibiotics by mycobacteria as well as low resistance to multiple drugs. Additionally, overexpression of pumps is the first step in developing clinical resistance, so it is essential to seek strategies to avoid the efflux effect of antibiotics. A plausible alternative is the use of efflux pump inhibitors such as verapamil or thioridazine, which assists in treatment with bedaquiline or rifampicin, key drugs for the control of drug-sensitive and multidrug-resistant tuberculosis.

Acknowledgements

Julieta Luna-Herrera is grateful for the support of the "Comisión de Operación y Fomento de Actividades Académicas" (COFAA), "Programa de Estímulos al Desempeño de los Investigadores" (EDI), Secretaria de Investigación y Posgrado (Project SIP-20240546), and "Sistema Nacional de Investigadoras e Investigadores" (SNII) of Secretaría de Ciencia, Humanidades, Tecnología e Innovación (SECIHTI). Karen Delgadillo-Gutiérrez is grateful for the support of the Secretaria de Investigación y Posgrado (Project SIP-20241170) and "Sistema Nacional de Investigadoras e Investigadores" (SNII) of SECIHTI. Axhell Aleid Cornejo-Báez holds a post-doctoral fellowship SECIHTI.

Conflict of interest

The authors declare no conflict of interest.

Author details

Julieta Luna-Herrera[1]*, Axhell Aleid Cornejo-Báez[1] and Karen Delgadillo-Gutiérrez[1,2]

1 Departamento de Inmunología, Escuela Nacional de Ciencias Biológicas, Instituto Politécnico Nacional, Ciudad de México, México

2 Secretaría de Ciencia, Humanidades, Tecnología e Innovación (SECIHTI), Ciudad de México, México

*Address all correspondence to: jlunah@ipn.mx

References

[1] Zhu Y, Liu Z, Peng L, Liu B, Wu K, Zhang M, et al. Evaluation of nucleotide MALDI-TOF-MS for the identification of *Mycobacterium* species. Frontiers in Cellular and Infection Microbiology. 2024;**14**:1335104

[2] Waman VP, Vedithi SC, Thomas SE, Bannerman BP, Munir A, Skwark MJ, et al. Mycobacterial genomics and structural bioinformatics: Opportunities and challenges in drug discovery. Emerging Microbes & Infections. 2019;**8**(1):109-118

[3] Raviglione MC, Snider DE Jr, Kochi A. Global epidemiology of tuberculosis. Morbidity and mortality of a worldwide epidemic. Journal of the American Medical Association. 1995;**273**(3):220-226

[4] Stokes RW, Norris-Jones R, Brooks DE, Beveridge TJ, Doxsee D, Thorson LM. The glycan-rich outer layer of the cell wall of *Mycobacterium tuberculosis* acts as an antiphagocytic capsule limiting the association of the bacterium with macrophages. Infection and Immunity. 2004;**72**(10):5676-5686

[5] Kalscheuer R, Palacios A, Anso I, Cifuente J, Anguita J, Jacobs WR, et al. The *Mycobacterium tuberculosis* capsule: A cell structure with key implications in pathogenesis. Biochemical Journal. 2019;**476**(14):1995-2016

[6] Dulberger CL, Rubin EJ, Boutte CC. The mycobacterial cell envelope — A moving target. Nature Reviews. Microbiology. 2020;**18**(1):47-59

[7] Nguyen L, Thompson CJ. Foundations of antibiotic resistance in bacterial physiology: The mycobacterial paradigm. Trends in Microbiology. 2006;**14**(7):304-312

[8] Ramaswamy S, Musser JM. Molecular genetic basis of antimicrobial agent resistance in *Mycobacterium tuberculosis*: 1998 update. Tubercle and Lung Disease. 1998;**79**(1):3-29

[9] Ebbensgaard AE, Løbner-Olesen A, Frimodt-Møller J. The role of efflux pumps in the transition from low-level to clinical antibiotic resistance. Antibiotics. 2020;**9**(12):855

[10] Gaurav A, Bakht P, Saini M, Pandey S, Pathania R. Role of bacterial efflux pumps in antibiotic resistance, virulence, and strategies to discover novel efflux pump inhibitors. Microbiology (N Y). 2023;**169**(5): 001333

[11] Van Bambeke F, Michot JM, Tulkens PM. Antibiotic efflux pumps in eukaryotic cells: Occurence and impact on antibiotic cellular pharmacokinetics, pharmacodynamics and toxicodynamics. Journal of Antimicrobial Chemotherapy. 2003;**51**(5):1067-1077

[12] Kabra R, Chauhan N, Kumar A, Ingale P, Singh S. Efflux pumps and antimicrobial resistance: Paradoxical components in systems genomics. Progress in Biophysics and Molecular Biology. 2019;**141**:15-24

[13] Biswas SS, Browne RB, Borah VV, Roy JD. In silico approach for phytocompound-based drug designing to fight efflux pump-mediated multidrug-resistant *Mycobacterium tuberculosis*. Applied Biochemistry and Biotechnology. 2021;**193**:1757-1779

[14] Hajiagha MN, Kafil HS. Efflux pumps and microbial biofilm formation. Infection, Genetics and Evolution. 2023;**112**:105459

[15] Silva PEA, Bigi F, De la Paz SM, Romano MI, Martín C, Cataldi A, et al. Characterization of P55, a multidrug efflux pump in *Mycobacterium bovis* and *Mycobacterium tuberculosis*. Antimicrobial Agents and Chemotherapy. 2001;**45**(3):800-804

[16] McGowen K, Funck T, Wang X, Zinga S, Wolf ID, Akusobi CC, et al. Efflux pumps and membrane permeability contribute to intrinsic antibiotic resistance in *Mycobacterium abscessus*. bioRxiv [Internet] 2024.08.23.609441. Available from: http://www.ncbi.nlm.nih.gov/pubmed/39229117

[17] Machado D, Lecorche E, Mougari F, Cambau E, Viveiros M. Insights on *Mycobacterium leprae* efflux pumps and their implications in drug resistance and virulence. Frontiers in Microbiology. 2018;**9**

[18] Black PA, Warren RM, Louw GE, Van Helden PD, Victor TC, Kana BD. Energy metabolism and drug efflux in *Mycobacterium tuberculosis*. Antimicrobial Agents and Chemotherapy. 2014;**58**:2491-2503

[19] Hassan KA, Liu Q, Elbourne LDH, Ahmad I, Sharples D, Naidu V, et al. Pacing across the membrane: The novel PACE family of efflux pumps is widespread in gram-negative pathogens. Research in Microbiology. 2018;**169**(7-8):450-454

[20] Laws M, Jin P, Rahman KM. Efflux pumps in *Mycobacterium tuberculosis* and their inhibition to tackle antimicrobial resistance. Trends in Microbiology. 2022;**30**:57-68

[21] de Oliveira MCB, Balan A. The ATP-binding cassette (ABC) transport systems in *Mycobacterium tuberculosis*: Structure, function, and possible targets for therapeutics. Biology. 2020;**9**:1-25

[22] Biswas SS, Roy JD. Prediction of structure of mycobacterial efflux pump protein Rv0194 and molecular dynamics simulation of the predicted structures. Biocatalysis and Agricultural Biotechnology. 2024;**61**:103381

[23] Nijland M, Lefebvre SN, Thangaratnarajah C, Slotboom DJ. Bidirectional ATP-driven transport of cobalamin by the mycobacterial ABC transporter BacA. Nature Communications. 2024;**15**(1):2626

[24] Kanji A, Hasan R, Ali A, Zaver A, Zhang Y, Imtiaz K, et al. Single nucleotide polymorphisms in efflux pumps genes in extensively drug resistant *Mycobacterium tuberculosis* isolates from Pakistan. Tuberculosis. 2017;**107**:20-30

[25] Pao SS, Paulsen IT, Saier MH. Major facilitator superfamily. Microbiology and Molecular Biology Reviews. 1998;**62**(1):1-34

[26] Fluman N, Bibi E. Bacterial multidrug transport through the lens of the major facilitator superfamily. Biochimica et Biophysica Acta (BBA) - Proteins and Proteomics. 2009;**1794**(5):738-747

[27] Pasqua M, Grossi M, Zennaro A, Fanelli G, Micheli G, Barras F, et al. The varied role of efflux pumps of the MFS family in the interplay of bacteria with animal and plant cells. Microorganisms. 2019;7(9):285

[28] Adhikary A, Biswal S, Ghosh AS. The putative major facilitator superfamily (MFS) protein named Rv1877 in *Mycobacterium tuberculosis* behaves as a multidrug efflux pump. Current Microbiology. 2022;**79**(11):324

[29] Bay DC, Rommens KL, Turner RJ. Small multidrug resistance proteins: A multidrug transporter family that

continues to grow. Biochimica et Biophysica Acta (BBA) - Biomembranes. 2008;**1778**(9):1814-1838

[30] Kermani AA, Macdonald CB, Burata OE, Ben Koff B, Koide A, Denbaum E, et al. The structural basis of promiscuity in small multidrug resistance transporters. Nature Communications. 2020;**11**(1):6064

[31] Burata OE, Yeh TJ, Macdonald CB, Stockbridge RB. Still rocking in the structural era: A molecular overview of the small multidrug resistance (SMR) transporter family. Journal of Biological Chemistry. 2022;**298**(10):102482

[32] Nikaido H. RND transporters in the living world. Research in Microbiology. 2018;**169**(7-8):363-371

[33] Sandhu P, Akhter Y. The drug binding sites and transport mechanism of the RND pumps from *Mycobacterium tuberculosis*: Insights from molecular dynamics simulations. Archives of Biochemistry and Biophysics. 2016;**592**:38-49

[34] Melly G, Purdy GE. MmpL proteins in physiology and pathogenesis of *M. Tuberculosis*. Microorganisms. 2019;**7**(3):70

[35] Domenech P, Reed MB, Barry CE. Contribution of the *Mycobacterium tuberculosis* MmpL protein family to virulence and drug resistance. Infection and Immunity. 2005;**73**(6):3492-3501

[36] Viljoen A, Dubois V, Girard-Misguich F, Blaise M, Herrmann J, Kremer L. The diverse family of MmpL transporters in mycobacteria: From regulation to antimicrobial developments developments. Molecular Microbiology. 2017;**104**(6):889-904

[37] Chalut C. MmpL transporter-mediated export of cell-wall associated lipids and siderophores in mycobacteria. Tuberculosis. 2016;**100**:32-45

[38] Sandhu P, Akhter Y. The internal gene duplication and interrupted coding sequences in the MmpL genes of *Mycobacterium tuberculosis*: Towards understanding the multidrug transport in an evolutionary perspective. International Journal of Medical Microbiology. 2015;**305**(3):413-423

[39] Lamichhane G, Tyagi S, Bishai WR. Designer arrays for defined mutant analysis to detect genes essential for survival of *Mycobacterium tuberculosis* in mouse lungs. Infection and Immunity. 2005;**73**(4):2533-2540

[40] Grzegorzewicz AE, Pham H, Gundi VAKB, Scherman MS, North EJ, Hess T, et al. Inhibition of mycolic acid transport across the *Mycobacterium tuberculosis* plasma membrane. Nature Chemical Biology. 2012;**8**(4):334-341

[41] Wells RM, Jones CM, Xi Z, Speer A, Danilchanka O, Doornbos KS, et al. Discovery of a Siderophore export system essential for virulence of *Mycobacterium tuberculosis*. PLoS Pathogens. 2013;**9**(1):e1003120

[42] Camacho LR, Constant P, Raynaud C, Lanéelle MA, Triccas JA, Gicquel B, et al. Analysis of the phthiocerol dimycocerosate locus of *Mycobacterium tuberculosis*. Evidence that this lipid is involved in the cell wall permeability barrier. Journal of Biological Chemistry. 2001;**276**(23):19845-19854

[43] Seeliger JC, Holsclaw CM, Schelle MW, Botyanszki Z, Gilmore SA, Tully SE, et al. Elucidation and chemical modulation of sulfolipid-1 biosynthesis in *Mycobacterium tuberculosis*. Journal of Biological Chemistry. 2012;**287**(11):7990-8000

[44] Mestre O, Hurtado-Ortiz R, Dos Vultos T, Namouchi A, Cimino M, Pimentel M, et al. High throughput phenotypic selection of *Mycobacterium tuberculosis* mutants with impaired resistance to reactive oxygen species identifies genes important for intracellular growth. PLoS One. 2013;**8**(1):e53486

[45] Ahmed M, Mackenzie J, Tezera L, Krause R, Truebody B, Garay-Baquero D, et al. *Mycobacterium tuberculosis* senses host interferon-γ via the membrane protein MmpL10. Communications Biology. 2022;**5**(1):1317

[46] Pacheco SA, Hsu FF, Powers KM, Purdy GE. MmpL11 protein transports mycolic acid-containing lipids to the mycobacterial Cell Wall and contributes to biofilm formation in *Mycobacterium smegmatis*. Journal of Biological Chemistry. 2013;**288**(33):24213-24222

[47] He X, Szewczyk P, Karyakin A, Evin M, Hong WX, Zhang Q, et al. Structure of a cation-bound multidrug and toxic compound extrusion transporter. Nature. 2010;**467**(7318):991-994

[48] Lu M. Structures of multidrug and toxic compound extrusion transporters and their mechanistic implications. Channels. 2016;**10**(2):88-100

[49] Mishra MN, Daniels L. Characterization of the MSMEG_2631 gene (mmp) encoding a multidrug and toxic compound extrusion (MATE) family protein in *Mycobacterium smegmatis* and exploration of its polyspecific nature using biolog phenotype MicroArray. Journal of Bacteriology. 2013;**195**(7):1610-1621

[50] Hassan KA, Jackson SM, Penesyan A, Patching SG, Tetu SG, Eijkelkamp BA, et al. Transcriptomic and biochemical analyses identify a family of chlorhexidine efflux proteins. National Academy of Sciences of the United States of America. 2013;**110**(50):20254-20259

[51] Hassan KA, Naidu V, Edgerton JR, Mettrick KA, Liu Q, Fahmy L, et al. Short-chain diamines are the physiological substrates of PACE family efflux pumps. National Academy of Sciences of the United States of America. 2019;**116**(36):18015-18020

[52] Bolla JR, Howes AC, Fiorentino F, Robinson CV. Assembly and regulation of the chlorhexidine-specific efflux pump AceI. National Academy of Sciences of the United States of America. 2020;**117**(29):17011-17018

[53] Danilchanka O, Mailaender C, Niederweis M. Identification of a novel multidrug efflux pump of *Mycobacterium tuberculosis*. Antimicrobial Agents and Chemotherapy. 2008;**52**(7):2503-2511

[54] Hasan Z, Razzak SA, Kanji A, Shakoor S, Hasan R. Efflux pump gene single-nucleotide variants associated with resistance in *Mycobacterium tuberculosis* isolates with discrepant drug genotypes. Journal of Global Antimicrobial Resistance. 2024;**38**:128-139

[55] Adhikary A, Chatterjee D, Ghosh AS. ABC superfamily transporter Rv1273c of *Mycobacterium tuberculosis* acts as a multidrug efflux pump. FEMS Microbiology Letters. 2023;**370**:fnad114

[56] Özgür D, Ersoy L, Ülger M, Tezcan Ülger S, Aslan G. Investigation of efflux pump genes in resistant *Mycobacterium tuberculosis* complex clinical isolates exposed to first line Antituberculosis drugs and verapamil combination. Mikrobiyoloji Bülteni. 2023;**57**(2):207-219

[57] Kumar Gupta A, Mohan Katoch V, Singh Chauhan D, Sharma R, Singh M, Venkatesan K, et al. Microarray analysis of efflux pump genes in multidrug-resistant *Mycobacterium tuberculosis* during stress induced by common anti-tuberculous drugs. Microbial Drug Resistance [Internet]. 2010;**16**(1):21-28. Available from: www.sanger.ac.uk=Projects=M_tuberculosis=Gene_list=

[58] Kardan-Yamchi J, Kazemian H, Haeili M, Harati AA, Amini S, Feizabadi MM. Expression analysis of 10 efflux pump genes in multidrug-resistant and extensively drug-resistant *Mycobacterium tuberculosis* clinical isolates. Journal of Global Antimicrobial Resistance. 2019;**17**:201-208

[59] Li X, Li P, Ruan C, xiang XL, Gu Y, Li J, et al. *Mycobacterium tuberculosis* Rv0191 is an efflux pump of major facilitator superfamily transporter regulated by Rv1353c. Archives of Biochemistry and Biophysics. 2019;**667**:59-66

[60] Vianna JS, Machado D, Ramis IB, Silva FP, Bierhals DV, Abril MA, et al. The contribution of efflux pumps in *Mycobacterium abscessus* complex resistance to clarithromycin. Antibiotics. 2019;**8**(3):153

[61] De Siena B, Campolattano N, D'Abrosca G, Russo L, Cantillon D, Marasco R, et al. Characterization of the *Mycobacterial* MSMEG-3762/63 efflux pump in *Mycobacterium smegmatis* drug efflux. Frontiers in Microbiology. 2020;**11**:575828

[62] Wang S, Wang K, Song K, Li P, Li D, Sun Y, et al. Structures of the essential efflux pump EfpA from *Mycobacterium tuberculosis* reveal the mechanisms of substrate transport and small-molecule inhibition. Research Square [Internet]. 2024:rs.3.rs-3740027. Available from: http://www.ncbi.nlm.nih.gov/pubmed/38260587

[63] Liu J, Shi W, Zhang S, Hao X, Maslov DA, Shur KV, et al. Mutations in efflux pump Rv1258c (tap) cause resistance to pyrazinamide, isoniazid, and streptomycin in M. Tuberculosis. Frontiers in Microbiology. 2019;**10**:216

[64] Ramón-García S, Mick V, Dainese E, Martín C, Thompson CJ, De Rossi E, et al. Functional and genetic characterization of the tap efflux pump in *Mycobacterium bovis* BCG. Antimicrobial Agents and Chemotherapy. 2012;**56**(4):2074-2083

[65] Buroni S, Manina G, Guglierame P, Pasca MR, Riccardi G, De Rossi E. LfrR is a repressor that regulates expression of the efflux pump LfrA in *Mycobacterium smegmatis*. Antimicrobial Agents and Chemotherapy. 2006;**50**(12):4044-4052

[66] De Rossi E, Blokpoel MCJ, Cantoni R, Branzoni M, Riccardi G, Young DB, et al. Molecular cloning and functional analysis of a novel tetracycline resistance determinant, tet(V), from *Mycobacterium smegmatis* [Internet]. Antimicrobial agents and chemotherapy. 1998;**42**(8):1931-1937. Available from: https://journals.asm.org/journal/aac

[67] Gupta AK, Reddy VP, Lavania M, Chauhan DS, Venkatesan K, Sharma VD, et al. jefA (Rv2459), a drug efflux gene in *Mycobacterium tuberculosis* confers resistance to isoniazid & ethambutol. Indian Journal of Medical Research. 2010;**132**(2):176-188

[68] Ramón-García S, Martín C, De Rossi E, Aínsa JA. Contribution of the Rv2333c efflux pump (the Stp protein) from *Mycobacterium tuberculosis* to intrinsic antibiotic resistance in *Mycobacterium bovis* BCG. Journal

of Antimicrobial Chemotherapy. 2007;**59**(3):544-547

[69] Gutiérrez AV, Richard M, Roquet-Banères F, Viljoen A, Kremer L. The TetR Family Transcription Factor MAB_2299c Regulates the Expression of Two Distinct MmpS-MmpL Efflux Pumps Involved in Cross-Resistance to Clofazimine and Bedaquiline in *Mycobacterium abscessus*. Antimicrobial agents and chemotherapy. 2019;**63**(10):e01000-19. Available from: https://journals.asm.org/journal/aac

[70] Narang A, Garima K, Porwal S, Bhandekar A, Shrivastava K, Giri A, et al. Potential impact of efflux pump genes in mediating rifampicin resistance in clinical isolates of *Mycobacterium tuberculosis* from India. PLoS One. 2019;**14**(9):e0223163

[71] Rindi L. Efflux pump inhibitors against nontuberculous mycobacteria. International Journal of Molecular Sciences. 2020;**21**(12):4191

[72] Allamyradov Y, Ben YJ, Kylychbekov S, Majidov I, Khuzhakulov Z, Er AY, et al. The role of efflux pump inhibitor in enhancing antimicrobial efficiency of Ag NPs and MB as an effective photodynamic therapy agent. Photodiagnosis and Photodynamic Therapy. 2024;**47**:104212

[73] Zhang L, Tian X, Sun L, Mi K, Wang R, Gong F, et al. Bacterial efflux pump inhibitors reduce antibiotic resistance. Pharmaceutics. 2024;**16**(2):170

[74] Pule CM, Sampson SL, Warren RM, Black PA, van Helden PD, Victor TC, et al. Efflux pump inhibitors: Targeting mycobacterial efflux systems to enhance TB therapy. Journal of Antimicrobial Chemotherapy. 2016;**71**(1):17-26

[75] Waditzer M, Bucar F. Flavonoids as inhibitors of bacterial efflux pumps. Molecules. 2021;**26**(22):6904

[76] Zhang S, Wang J, Ahn J. Advances in the discovery of efflux pump inhibitors as novel potentiators to control antimicrobial-resistant pathogens. Antibiotics. 2023;**12**(9):1417

[77] Viveiros M, Martins M, Rodrigues L, Machado D, Couto I, Ainsa J, et al. Inhibitors of mycobacterial efflux pumps as potential boosters for anti-tubercular drugs. Expert Review of Anti-Infective Therapy. 2012;**10**(9):983-998

[78] Song L, Wu X. Development of efflux pump inhibitors in antituberculosis therapy. International Journal of Antimicrobial Agents. 2016;**47**(6):421-429

[79] Martin A, Bouyakoub Y, Soumillion K, Mantu EN, Colmant A, Rodriguez-Villalobos H. Targeting Bedaquiline mycobacterial efflux pump to potentially enhance therapy in *Mycobacterium Abscessus*. The International Journal of Mycobacteriology. 2020;**9**(1):71-75

[80] Sellamuthu S, Bhat MF, Kumar A, Singh SK. Phenothiazine: A better scaffold against tuberculosis. Mini-Reviews in Medicinal Chemistry. 2018;**18**(17):1442-1451

[81] Sessa L, Concilio S, Marrafino F, Sarkar A, Diana R, Piotto S. Theoretical investigation of hydroxylated analogues of valinomycin as potassium transporter. Computational Biology and Chemistry. 2023;**106**:107936

[82] Puk K, Guz L. Effect of alkaloid berberine on the susceptibility of nontuberculous mycobacteria to antibiotics. Polish Journal of Veterinary Sciences. 2022;**25**(3):479-481

[83] Solnier J, Martin L, Bhakta S, Bucar F. Flavonoids as novel efflux pump inhibitors and antimicrobials against

both environmental and pathogenic intracellular mycobacterial species. Molecules. 2020;**25**(3):734

[84] Webber MA. The importance of efflux pumps in bacterial antibiotic resistance. Journal of Antimicrobial Chemotherapy. 2003;**51**(1):9-11

[85] Kanji A, Hasan R, Hasan Z. Efflux pump as alternate mechanism for drug resistance in *Mycobacterium tuberculosis*. Indian Journal of Tuberculosis. 2019;**66**(1):20-25

[86] Li XZ, Livermore DM, Nikaido H. Role of efflux pump(s) in intrinsic resistance of *Pseudomonas aeruginosa*: Resistance to tetracycline, chloramphenicol, and norfloxacin. Antimicrobial Agents and Chemotherapy. 1994;**38**(8):1732-1741

[87] Andries K, Villellas C, Coeck N, Thys K, Gevers T, Vranckx L, et al. Acquired resistance of *Mycobacterium tuberculosis* to Bedaquiline. PLoS One. 2014;**9**(7):e102135

[88] Du D, Wang-Kan X, Neuberger A, van Veen HW, Pos KM, Piddock LJV, et al. Multidrug efflux pumps: structure, function and regulation. Nature Reviews. Microbiology. 2018;**16**(9):523-539

[89] Srikrishna G, Gupta S, Dooley KE, Bishai WR. Can the addition of verapamil to Bedaquiline-containing regimens improve tuberculosis treatment outcomes? A novel approach to optimizing TB treatment. Future Microbiology. 2015;**10**(8):1257-1260

[90] Shafer WM, Yu EW, Rouquette-Loughlin C, Golparian D, Jerse AE, Unemo M. Efflux pumps in *Neisseria gonorrhoeae*: Contributions to antimicrobial resistance and virulence. In: Efflux-Mediated Antimicrobial Resistance in Bacteria. Cham: Springer International Publishing; 2016. pp. 439-469

[91] Goossens SN, Sampson SL, Van RA. Mechanisms of drug-induced tolerance in *Mycobacterium tuberculosis*. Clinical Microbiology Reviews. 2020;**34**(1):e00141-20. DOI: 10.1128/CMR.00141-20

[92] Machado D, Couto I, Perdigão J, Rodrigues L, Portugal I, Baptista P, et al. Contribution of efflux to the emergence of isoniazid and multidrug resistance in *Mycobacterium tuberculosis*. PLoS One. 2012;**7**(4):e34538

[93] Schmalstieg AM, Srivastava S, Belkaya S, Deshpande D, Meek C, Leff R, et al. The antibiotic resistance arrow of time: Efflux pump induction is a general first step in the evolution of mycobacterial drug resistance. Antimicrobial Agents and Chemotherapy. 2012;**56**(9):4806-4815

[94] Jang S. AcrAB-TolC, a major efflux pump in gram negative bacteria: Toward understanding its operation mechanism. BMB Reports. 2023;**56**(6):326-334

[95] El Meouche I, Dunlop MJ. Heterogeneity in efflux pump expression predisposes antibiotic-resistant cells to mutation. Science (1979). 2018;**362**(6415):686-690

[96] Bhattacharyya S, Bhattacharyya M, Pfannenstiel DM, Nandi AK, Hwang Y, Ho K, et al. Efflux-linked accelerated evolution of antibiotic resistance at a population edge. Molecular Cell. 2022;**82**(22):4368-4385.e6

[97] Du Toit A. Efflux pumps, fitness and virulence. Nature Reviews. Microbiology. 2017;**15**(9):512-513

[98] Olivares, Pacheco J, Alvarez-Ortega C, Alcalde Rico M, Martínez JL.

Metabolic compensation of fitness costs is a general outcome for antibiotic-resistant *Pseudomonas aeruginosa* mutants overexpressing efflux pumps. MBio. 2017;**8**(4):e00500

[99] Olivares J, Álvarez-Ortega C, Martinez JL. Metabolic compensation of fitness costs associated with overexpression of the multidrug efflux pump MexEF-OprN in *Pseudomonas aeruginosa*. Antimicrobial Agents and Chemotherapy. 2014;**58**(7):3904-3913

[100] Singha B, Murmu S, Nair T, Rawat RS, Sharma AK, Soni V. Metabolic rewiring of *Mycobacterium tuberculosis* upon drug treatment and antibiotics resistance. Metabolites. 2024;**14**(1):63

[101] Andersson DI, Levin BR. The biological cost of antibiotic resistance. Current Opinion in Microbiology. 1999;**2**(5):489-493

[102] Davies AP, Billington OJ, Bannister BA, Weir WRC, McHugh TD, Gillespie SH. Comparison of fitness of two isolates of *Mycobacterium tuberculosis*, one of which had developed multi-drug resistance during the course of treatment. Journal of Infection. 2000;**41**(2):184-187

[103] Alame, Emane AK, Guo X, Takiff HE, Liu S. Drug resistance, fitness and compensatory mutations in *Mycobacterium tuberculosis*. Tuberculosis. 2021;**129**:102091

[104] Comas I, Borrell S, Roetzer A, Rose G, Malla B, Kato-Maeda M, et al. Whole-genome sequencing of rifampicin-resistant *Mycobacterium tuberculosis* strains identifies compensatory mutations in RNA polymerase genes. Nature Genetics. 2012;**44**(1):106-110

[105] de Vos M, Müller B, Borrell S, Black PA, van Helden PD, Warren RM, et al. Putative compensatory mutations in the rpoC gene of Rifampin-resistant *Mycobacterium tuberculosis* are associated with ongoing transmission. Antimicrobial Agents and Chemotherapy. 2013;**57**(2):827-832

[106] Stefan MA, Ugur FS, Garcia GA. Source of the fitness defect in Rifamycin-resistant *Mycobacterium tuberculosis* RNA polymerase and the mechanism of compensation by mutations in the β′ subunit. Antimicrobial Agents and Chemotherapy. 2018;**62**(6):e00164-18

[107] Briffotaux J, Huang W, Wang X, Gicquel B. MmpS5/MmpL5 as an efflux pump in *Mycobacterium* species. Tuberculosis. 2017;**107**:13-19

[108] Lamut A, Peterlin Mašič L, Kikelj D, Tomašič T. Efflux pump inhibitors of clinically relevant multidrug resistant bacteria. Medicinal Research Reviews. 2019;**39**(6):2460-2504

[109] Arefanian H, Koti L, Sindhu S, Ahmad R, Al Madhoun A, Al-Mulla F. Verapamil chronicles: Advances from cardiovascular to pancreatic β-cell protection. Frontiers in Pharmacology. 2023;**14**:1322148

[110] Adams KN, Takaki K, Connolly LE, Wiedenhoft H, Winglee K, Humbert O, et al. Drug tolerance in replicating mycobacteria mediated by a macrophage-induced efflux mechanism. Cell. 2011;**145**(1):39-53

[111] Gupta S, Tyagi S, Almeida DV, Maiga MC, Ammerman NC, Bishai WR. Acceleration of tuberculosis treatment by adjunctive therapy with verapamil as an efflux inhibitor. American Journal of Respiratory and Critical Care Medicine. 2013;**188**(5):600-607

[112] Padmapriyadarsini C, Szumowski JD, Akbar N, Shanmugasundaram P, Jain A, Bathragiri M, et al. A dose-finding study to guide use of verapamil as an adjunctive therapy in tuberculosis. Clinical Pharmacology and Therapeutics. 2024;**115**(2):324-332

[113] Kimbell I, Overall JE, Winkelman GW, Hughes WM. Comparison of thioridazine and chlorpromazine in doctor's choice research design. Clinical Pharmacology and Therapeutics. 1971;**12**(5):825-832

[114] Amaral L, Viveiros M. Why thioridazine in combination with antibiotics cures extensively drug-resistant *Mycobacterium tuberculosis* infections. International Journal of Antimicrobial Agents. 2012;**39**:376-380

[115] Amaral L, Viveiros M. Thioridazine: A non-antibiotic drug highly effective, in combination with first line anti-tuberculosis drugs, against any form of antibiotic resistance of *Mycobacterium tuberculosis* due to its multi-mechanisms of action. Antibiotics. 2017;**6**(1):3

[116] Abbate E, Vescovo M, Natiello M, Cufré M, García A, Montaner PG, et al. Successful alternative treatment of extensively drug-resistant tuberculosis in Argentina with a combination of linezolid, moxifloxacin and thioridazine. Journal of Antimicrobial Chemotherapy. 2012;**67**(2):473-477

Chapter 5

Antigen Processing Pathways in *Mycobacterium tuberculosis* Pathogenesis and Links to Clinical Presentation

Karolina D. Witt

Abstract

Mycobacterium tuberculosis (Mtb) is an intracellular pathogen that has co-evolved with humans and developed various decoy strategies to survive in hostile environments by manipulating host immunity to its advantage. This occurs through selective antigen presentation at the cellular level, induction of dysfunctional immune responses, and a clinical latency period that hampers active surveillance of disease transmission. The spectrum of clinical symptoms is a function of immune responses and may, but does not necessarily, correlate directly with disease burden. This chapter will explore the biology of *Mycobacterium tuberculosis,* focusing on selected genes and their products that are crucial in host-pathogen interactions, which subsequently result in the clinical presentation of tuberculosis (TB). It will look at the bacilli's intracellular location, its antigens' release and presentation, their processing pathways, immune responses, and granuloma formation. Both pulmonary and extrapulmonary clinical presentations are presented, including the destructive role of inflammation in the disease. The chapter will also briefly mention *Mtb* genes used in rapid clinical diagnostics and the role of selected TB antigens in the design of new vaccines.

Keywords: *Mycobacterium tuberculosis*, intracellular pathogen, antigen presentation, host-pathogen interactions, latent infection, granuloma, inflammation, pulmonary tuberculosis, extrapulmonary tuberculosis

1. Introduction

Global impact. *Mycobacterium tuberculosis (Mtb)* is the causative agent of tuberculosis (TB), an infectious disease responsible for 7.5 million newly diagnosed cases, 10.6 million overall TB cases worldwide, and 1.3 million deaths annually [1].

Epidemiology and risk factors. This potentially preventable and usually curable disease remains one of the leading causes of death from a single infectious pathogen. While not an opportunistic pathogen *per se, Mtb* disproportionately affects socially disadvantaged populations, with an endemic focus in low- and middle-income countries. In other regions, TB is concentrated within migrant communities, prisoners, and travellers, but also affects individuals with alcohol dependence, exposure to smoke or open-fire cooking, homelessness, or other forms of social deprivation. Living in crowded households in close proximity to the infectious individuals correlates with higher TB incidence [2] through intense *Mtb* transmission within the households. Limited access to healthcare through restricted financial resources or an insufficient number of qualified personnel regionally widens TB knowledge gaps and contributes to TB incidence. [3] TB is also more frequent in people living with HIV and in immunocompromised persons [4].

Evolutionary Adaptations of *Mtb*. The evolutionary success of *Mtb* is often attributed to its prevalence in disadvantaged communities. However, this simplification overlooks the myriad ways of interactions between the pathogen and its host, where persistence and clinical latency are more common outcomes than epidemic outbreaks. Due to these attributes, *Mtb* silently infects approximately 20–25% of the world's population, and its strains exhibit genomic variations that reflect close adaptation to local host communities [5, 6]. Pulmonary tuberculosis, the primary transmission route for *Mtb,* occurs when the bacilli are released in small aerosol droplets [7] through coughing, passing into the lower respiratory tract of a recipient where the tissue-resident macrophages are present. Clinically symptomatic infection is a relatively rare outcome of this initial encounter. Ghon focus [8] is traditionally recognised as the site of primary infection; areas of calcified tissues and cavities can be diagnosed anywhere on a routine chest X-ray, but in most cases, it is impossible to link this entity to any clinically identifiable episode of the disease in the patient's medical history. On the other side, this primary site has the propensity to seed bacilli into lymph nodes and, via haematogenous routes, to reactivate later at any site.

Host-pathogen interactions. Following the phagocytosis of *Mtb* by macrophages, the pathogen triggers a number of host pathways that delay the process of phagosome-lysosome fusion and pathogen degradation [9]. This delay enables selective antigen presentation on the macrophage surface, attracting other immune cells but, at the same time, sequestering the bacilli within the macrophage cell. During this process, the acquisition of lipids reduces the metabolic activity of *Mtb,* which then enters into a persistent, dormant state [10].

Immunological Mechanisms. Immune responses during primary infection involve alveolar M2 macrophages, which predominantly rely on focused, respiratory chain-driven reactive-oxygen species (ROS) responses to target the intracellular invader. For *Mtb* to survive and disseminate while still in the relatively vulnerable stage of active replication, it needs to be transferred to blood-derived M1 macrophages and dendritic cells, which transport the bacilli to local lymph nodes. These cells are more proficient at stimulating host immune responses but are also more susceptible to succumbing to the bacilli, dying through apoptosis, which in turn stimulates antigen presentation. This pathogen passaging between macrophages initiates the formation of granulomas, accompanied by an influx of neutrophils and T cells, which collectively seclude and shield Mtb. When granuloma formation fails—either due to pathogen hypervirulence [11], weakened host immunity, or co-infection with HIV [12]—miliary TB can develop. This form of TB, characterised by a disseminated pattern of granular densities, results in clinically symptomatic disease; however, granulomatous pulmonary cavitation is usually a more infectious TB presentation.

2. Innate immunity: Intracellular events following infection

Alveolar macrophages serve as the first port of entry and primary host for *Mtb*, killing most of the bacilli while also sheltering their persistent forms [13]. The process of phagosomal uptake involves a range of cell receptors, including pattern recognition receptors (PRRs), Toll-like receptors (TLRs), C-type lectin receptors, scavenger receptors, nucleotide-binding oligomerisation domain (NOD)-like receptors, and complement receptors for bacilli opsonised with immunoglobulins [14]. Many of these receptors promote phagocytosis but not necessarily pathogen eradication—one of the decoy strategies *Mtb* uses to survive within its host [15].

The arrest of phagosome maturation is an important stage in the *Mtb* life cycle [**Figure 1**]. *Mtb* influences the acidification of the phagosome in the early phase of infection by preventing the tethering of host H^+-ATPase to the *Mtb*-containing vacuole with its tyrosine phosphatase *PtpA*, preventing luminal acidification and stabilising its pH at 6.3–6.5 [16]. The early phagosome undergoes a series of encounters

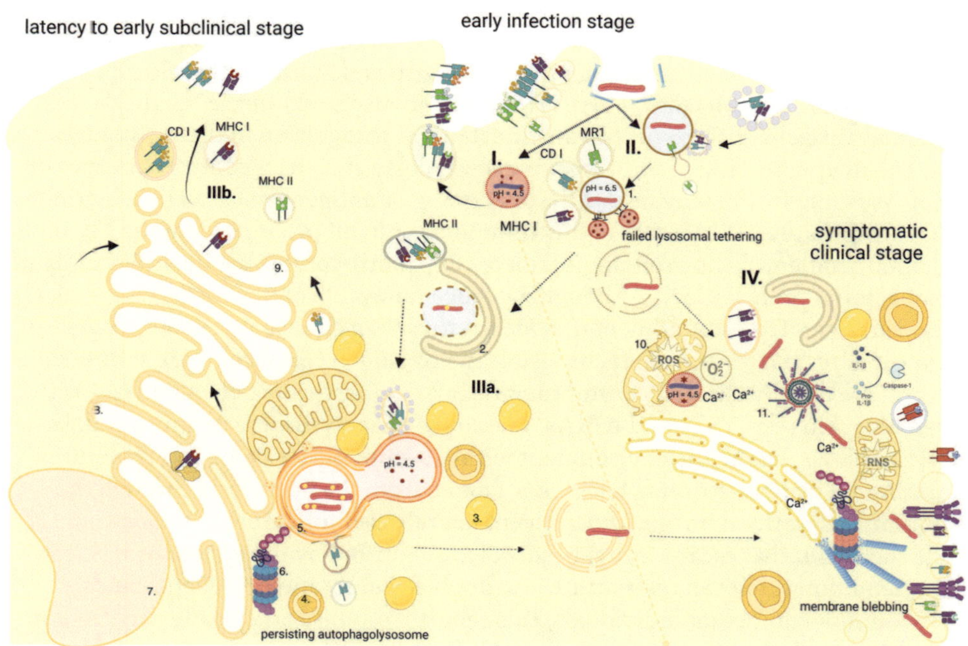

Figure 1.
Mtb life cycle and antigen processing during the course of the intracellular stage of Mtb infection. The figure represents stages of phagocytosed bacilli (pathways are time- and site-specific). (I) The phagolysosome disables the pathogen while presented antigens are derived from fragmented dead bacilli. (II) Persistent phagosomes where fusion with lysosome was blocked successfully by the bacilli: presented antigens are virulence factors released by live Mtb. (III) Autophagolysosomes with persistent latent bacilli: presented antigens are scanty and a by-product of pathogen-host cellular organelle interactions: (IIIa) stage of autophagosome nucleation initiation and (IIIb) a stage of persisting autophagolysosome communicating with Endoplasmic Reticulum (ER) and endosomes. (IV) Cytosol bacilli—irreversible destruction of cell innate defence, generalised disruption of cell functions (damaged mitochondria, activation of inflammasomes), and likely progress to cell death. Dashed arrows represent pathogen transition; solid arrows represent sources of the antigen. Cellular structures annotation: 1. Phagosome 2. Double-layer membrane systems 3. Lipid droplets 4. Peroxisome 5. Autophagolysosome 6. Ubiquitin-Proteasome system 7. Nucleus 8. Endoplasmic Reticulum (ER) 9. Golgi system 10. Mitochondrion 11. Inflammasome. Created with BioRender.com.

with other intracellular endocytic organelles to acquire various molecules, including MHC-I and MHC-II receptors. Mycobacterial Man LAM blocks the transport of acidic cargo from the trans-Golgi network [13], while its protein kinase G (pknG) is involved in malfunction interplay between Rab5 and Rab7 acquisition, directly interfering with the Rab7-associated signalling process, which results in preventing phagosome-lysosome fusion, favouring pathogen survival inside macrophages [17, 18]. This temporary blocking effect is eventually overcome by IFN-γ activated macrophages, immune responses to mycobacterial early conserved immunodominant epitopes of the *Esx* secretion system triggering a pH drop to 5.0 in the phagolysosome. However, the time gained allows *Mtb* to alter its ability to use diverse carbon sources, activating the glyoxylate shunt [19] and storage of cholesterol and neutral lipids like triacylglycerols (TAG) in lipid droplets [10], followed by the mycobacteria entry into the dormant phase and starting latency phase of TB infection.

During the early infection stage, *Mtb*-containing phagosomes fuse with specialised MHC-II receptors containing endosomes, recycling endosomes containing MHC-I molecules endocytosed from the cell surface, and trafficking nonclassical MR1 molecules from the trans-Golgi network [20]. Mtb antigens, compartmentalised in different cellular regions, are loaded onto MHC molecules either directly or after initial processing, which determines peptide length and assists in their loading onto MHC-I or MHC-II molecules. There is limited knowledge about the "quality" of presented antigens with respect to the infected cell recognition in the early stages after bacilli uptake. However, pathogen-caused delay and strict control over the timing of lysosome fusion may favour the processing of antigens released by live bacilli. These antigens are likely small, highly immunodominant proteins from the *Esx* family [21] and members of the proline-glutamate (PE) motif-containing PE-PPE family of mycobacterial proteins [22]. Although evidence for events in this earliest stage of TB infection comes from experimental models rather than clinical cases, they represent the stage of primary infection focus visible in imaging as Ghon complex at its resolution and are usually clinically asymptomatic but diagnostically detectable in positive tuberculin skin test (TST) and IGRAs. The single phagolysosome membrane does not persist for long. The acidic environment within eventually weakens and punctures it, facilitated by pore-forming bacilli *Esx* factors from the bacilli and through the membrane oxidative damage. *Mtb* antigens are released for cytosolic processing [21], while the bacilli that escape into the cytosol are captured by the system of intracellular membranes that can restructure into double-membrane autophagosomes.

In immunocompetent individuals, this cellular response is typically sufficient to either destroy the bacilli via autophagosome-lysosome fusion and pathogen destruction in the low pH environment or at least compartmentalise the bacilli away from other organelles, inducing the pathogen's entry into a dormant state of latency. While it was reported that bacillary resuscitation may happen many years after initial infection, there is also evidence indicating the incubation period for the development of active TB from the first evidence of exposure in the form of tuberculin skin test [TST] conversion rarely exceeds two years [23].

As Mtb-containing autophagolysosomes persist intracellularly, the spectrum of presented molecules shifts from highly immunodominant proteins to subdominant proteins and lipids involved in the range of bacterial metabolic processes. There is an established balance of secreted pathogen antigens with molecular signal sequences that penetrate the autophagosome membranes to influence host metabolism, respiration [24], and antigen processing [25] before the bacilli eventually succumb to the inhospitable environment of activated macrophages, which characterises resolution of infection and reverse conversion of TST. Interestingly, these subdominant antigens are believed to elicit more effective immune responses and longer immune memory. Examples of these proteins include *DnaK, CpsY, Erm37, Eis, PPE18, PPE2,* and *LprG* [26–32].

Periodically, or upon triggers such as a drop in immune surveillance due to unrelated diseases, immunocompromise due to malnutrition, poor glucose control, or repetitive exposure to TB, resuscitating and actively replicating bacilli puncture membranes to escape back to the cytosol. The process of bacilli separation into autophagosomes may repeat again, or infected macrophages may undergo remodelling and fuse into Langhans multinucleate giant cells, potentially facilitated by phenolic glycolipids from the bacilli [33]. The disruption of intracellular membrane continuity can also lead to cell death through apoptosis, necrosis [34], pyroptosis [35], or ferroptosis [36]—each with distinct characteristics that determine the degree of antigen presentation to other phagocytes and antigen-presenting cells. Type I IFN, induced by the cytosolic DNA sensor cGAS activated by mycobacterial DNA, is associated with decreased glycolysis, mitochondrial stress, the production of mitochondrial ROS, and the release of mitochondrial DNA. This further escalates type I IFN signalling and leads to the collapse of cellular respiration, contributing to Mtb pathogenesis and the bacilli's exit from the host cell [37, 38]. Clinically symptomatic stage of the disease starts when bacilli activity and dissemination escalate to break through the host barriers.

3. Development of granuloma

Alveolar macrophages, the initial host cells for *Mtb,* are not the only players in tuberculosis pathogenesis. Directly infected macrophages and secondary phagocytes, which engulf infected cells, form the initial granuloma aggregate. This compact structure includes diverse macrophage forms, such as epithelioid-like cells, foam cells, and multinucleated giant cells, whose development is driven by platelets [39]. As the infection progresses, other immune cells are attracted to the infection site, while the infected macrophage migrates to mediastinal lymph nodes and lymphatic vessels [40]. The granuloma-forming cells include granulocytes with innate lymphoid cells [41] and natural killer (NK) cells, and dendritic cells interspersed among them, stromal compartment of fibroblasts, Langhans giant cells, myeloid-derived suppressor cells [MDSCs] [42], epithelial cells, and lymphocytes, which form the outer cuff of the granuloma, sealing it into a self-contained unit [43]. NK cells are effector cells with cytotoxic properties that respond to early stages of infection without previous antigen exposure reacting instead to subtle changes in MHC-I presentation on the cell surface by the action of activating or inhibitory killer-cell immunoglobulin-like receptors (KIRs) and natural killer (NK) receptors, respectively [44]. They are also endowed with non-specific innate memory trained through epigenetic reprogramming [45]. Dendritic cells and B cells participate in local antigen presentation and deliver antigens to the lymph nodes [46]. Within 2–3 months of *Mtb* infection, the granuloma grows into a 2–4 mm spherical structure that restrains and contains infection rather than eliminating it, minimising pathogen spread when complete sterilisation is not possible outright.

At the molecular level, the necrotic centre of the granuloma contains antimicrobial peptides, effectors of tumour necrosis factor α (TNF-α) and IFN-γ signalling pathways, ROS, reactive nitrogen species (RNS), and enzymes that produce 5-lipoxygenase (5-LOX) derivatives [47], such as leukotriene B4 (LTB4), an important regulator of TNF-α [35]. In contrast, the cellular periphery of the necrotising granuloma or throughout the solid granulomas exhibits a signature of higher levels of cyclooxygenase COX-1/2 derivatives, such as prostaglandin E2 (PGE2). Granulomas within the lungs develop heterogeneously—histologically, there may be early, mature, solid, calcifying, necrotising, or even liquifying with cavities in advanced stages [36]. The gradient of centrally focused proinflammatory highly reactive molecules to more anti-inflammatory cuff with the presence of high levels of CD4 T lymphocytes is vital for effective barrier formation and functionality to maintain equilibrium in the immune responses and ongoing activation of APCs.

Cellular immunity in the form of localised delayed-type hypersensitivity reaction to Mtb antigens like cord factor (trehalose 6,6′-dimycolate, TDM) [48] is a hallmark of TB infection and contributes to granuloma development. The interaction between T cells and infected macrophages induces IFN-γ production of T cells and activated macrophages that secrete cytokines and chemokines. These immune signals, including host matrix metalloproteinases (MMPs), initially facilitate chemotaxis of neutrophils, fibroblasts, and monocytes to the granuloma; however, soon the excess of inflammatory mediators leads to non-antigen-specific anergy of overstimulated immune cells and remodelling of the lung tissue with loss of its original function.

In granulomas progressing to active disease, a distinct $CD8^+$ T cell signature correlates with a higher disease burden [49]. The most distinctive feature of necrotic granulomas is the presence of caseum, a soft mass of necrotic macrophages, along with acellular lipid-loaded debris and free, often drug-recalcitrant, persisting acid-fast bacilli [50, 51]. High lipid load enhances the virulence of cord factor and pathogen activity [52]. $CD8^+$ T cells and activated NK cell signatures are associated with high microbial burden and cavitating disease in tuberculosis and respond rapidly to the anti-tuberculosis treatment [53, 54].

Depending on the size and location of the granuloma, its rupture may lead to the release of its content into the airways, leading to periods of intensified cough and transmission of actively replicating *Mtb*, with occasional haemoptysis depending on the vascular composition of the surrounding destroyed tissue. Conversely, in mature granulomas where sterilisation of the bacilli occurs, an immunoregulatory phenotype dominates with a higher prevalence of epithelial cells, fibroblasts, and cells involved in angiogenesis, indicating tissue remodelling and repair. However, in the context of pulmonary TB, this remodelling does not typically restore the alveolar structure and respiratory function of the lungs.

4. Acquired immunity

While the exact correlates of protective responses in TB are not fully understood [55], $CD4^+$ and $CD8^+$ T cells play crucial roles in cellular immunity to TB, and both HLA class I and II antigen presentation to $CD8^+$ T cells has been linked to both susceptibility and severity of the disease [56, 57]. $CD4^+$ and $CD8^+$ T cells are primarily responsible for the initial control of infection at the site by interacting directly with antigen-presenting cells (APCs) and producing IFN-γ and other cytokines. They are also essential for the development of T cell memory.

Antigen-specific $CD4^+$ responses appear early in the form of immune responses to early Mtb antigens. These cells are frequently rendered anergic by immunodominant TB antigens of key virulence factors, and soon the $CD4^+$ population becomes more populated with IL-10-secreting $CD4^+$ regulatory T cells (Tregs), which further drives this anergy [58, 59]. The phenomenon of T cell anergy is complex, involving mitochondrial activity, mass, and cellular metabolism. A study on the diabetic drug metformin showed that improving host metabolic fitness increases resistance to Mtb infection [60]. Functionally active CD4$^+$ T cells secrete three key cytokines in response to Mtb antigens: IL-2, IFN-γ, and TNF-α. The ability to secrete these cytokines divides T cells into mono- or polyfunctional cells. Although polyfunctional cells, which secrete multiple cytokines, are deemed to be superior effectors with a higher proliferating capacity, this finding comes from studies focused on vaccine responses rather than natural infection. Conversely, it is well-known that impairment of TNF-α responses through blocking monoclonal antibodies used in inflammatory diseases heightens the risk of progression to active TB disease [61, 62]. Studies of polyfunctionality in mycobacteria-specific T cell responses indicated a higher frequency of TNF-α, IFN-γ, and IL-2 secretion in latent disease [63], active diseases [50], or no association at all [64]. These differences could point either toward subtle changes in the granularity of TB staging or population-dependent factors, such as genetic background or environmental exposure that modulate these immune responses.

The role of antigen-specific CD8$^+$ T cells as correlates of protection remains unclear, both in natural infection and in vaccine responses. These CD8$^+$ T cells are detectable in both active and latent TB [65, 66]. Upon activation, CD8$^+$ T cells produce cytotoxic granules containing granulysin, granzyme A and B, and perforin, which are discharged into immune synapses upon direct contact with target cells. They also produce Th1-type cytokines, including IFNγ, TNFα and IL-2. Despite their potent effector functions, CD8$^+$ responses in TB are discordant. Upon initial infection, CD8+ T cells serve as sensors of high mycobacterial burden, but given *Mtb*'s ability to infect in small numbers, these cells may not be sufficiently activated. In chronic TB, CD8$^+$ T cells can become functionally anergic in granuloma, with reduced expression of cytotoxic molecules compared to those at peripheral sites [67].

With advancements in mass cytometry and multiparametric flow cytometry, the complexity of immune responses to TB is becoming more recognised. NK cells, B cells and invariant natural killer T (iNKT) cells, mucosa-associated invariant T cells (MAIT) and γδ T cells [68], some also endowed with limited residential memory functions have been detected at sites of the disease while the proportion of monocyte-to-lymphocyte and neutrophil-to-lymphocyte ratios characterises the active TB disease. Altogether, these immune cells form a TB immune signature in blood and at peripheral tissues, and they recognise a wide range of protein antigens, as well as Mtb mycoketides, mycolates [69], glycolipids, lipopolysaccharides, and riboflavin derivatives of *Mtb* metabolism [70].

5. Clinical presentation in tuberculosis

Infection with *Mtb* confers an average 5–10% lifetime risk of developing tuberculosis [71, 72], with the majority of this risk occurring within the first 2 years after infection. Statistical modelling of large population studies has shown that this risk can be further split into a higher proportion of individuals developing the minimal subclinical disease, while a smaller minority progresses to a full range of clinical symptoms [73]. Exact estimates of these proportions may vary regionally, reflecting recurrences and relapse in settings with very high TB incidence [74].

Infectious droplets are the primary route of TB transmission. These droplets, typically smaller than 100 microns, contain 1–10 *Mtb* bacilli each [7] and are propelled at speeds up to 50 mph during coughing. However, coughing is not a prerequisite for TB transmission, as bacilli can also be transmitted during close contact while sleeping, speaking loudly, or singing [75]. Effective transmission depends on the ability of *Mtb* to infect even with a small number of bacilli that bypass the heavily colonised upper respiratory airways and reach the sparsely populated small bronchioles and alveoli, where alveolar macrophages reside.

The classification of TB clinical presentation has evolved in the last decade, moving away from the binary division of latent infection and active disease that was established with the introduction of the first antibiotic treatments. Microbiological confirmation became a prerequisite for treatment, facilitating the development of programmatic TB management, including contact tracing. However, gaps remain, especially regarding under-recognised diseases in individuals not reporting TB symptoms. These individuals may have subclinical TB and could benefit from preventative treatment, particularly in the presence of other risk factors, but with consideration for the risk of drug resistance development in affected populations. Resistance to first-line drugs, rifampicin, and isoniazid, which constitute both preventative and first-line treatment, can be diagnosed using rapid diagnostic tests, but levofloxacin is so far the only alternative in preventative treatment for multidrug-resistant TB [MDR-TB] [76]. Even for drug-susceptible TB bacilli, polypharmacotherapy is required. Drug resistance is defined as resistance to at least one first-line TB drug, typically isoniazid or rifampicin. Multidrug resistance [MDR] involves resistance to both of these drugs, requiring treatment with second-line drugs. Programmatic TB control helps identify individuals infected with TB [77]. In low-burden countries, there is a shift away from using a positive interferon-gamma release assays (IGRA) test alone as the sole indication for latent TB treatment unless there are associated risk factors [78]. Predictors of TB morbidity include factors such as the *Mt*b strain and its virulence, environmental and social factors, genetic and immune susceptibility, comorbidities, and concurrent treatments. Additionally, infectiousness is linked to the bacterial load and the metabolic activity of *Mtb*. High-throughput computational data analytics are needed to develop population-specific algorithms to identify subclinically infected TB individuals, who are infectious [79]. A two-stage process involving PCR-based *Mtb* detection, followed by sputum culture-positive bacteriological confirmation in pre-treatment samples, even in the absence of clinical symptoms, could represent a future standard. Preventative treatment with two drugs (rifampicin and isoniazid) could begin upon receiving PCR results, with escalation to full treatment after bacteriological confirmation. This approach could help address issues related to TB stigma and the challenges of collecting blood samples while maintaining similar cost-effectiveness. However, it is highly dependent on the accessibility of PCR-based diagnostics. Such targeted preventative treatment may interrupt transmission chains, improve health outcomes, and have minimal impact on the development of drug resistance. The current approach to TB staging has returned, to some extent, to a pre-antibiotic era of descriptive disease classification. It uses three key disease dimensions: pathology, infectivity, and clinical symptoms/signs [80]. These dimensions, in various combinations, define five distinct states of TB as outlined in **Table 1**.

This approach reflects in more detail the complex interdependencies and dynamics between TB disease incidence, sputum-smear-positive asymptomatic cases, and clinically symptomatic TB. Imaging diagnostics, from first-line chest X-rays to CT, MRI, and less commonly available PET-CT, allow for screening and staging TB pathology. While primary TB typically forms granulomas, post-primary TB lesions

Staging	Macroscopic pathology	Infectious	TB symptoms and signs
Mtb infection	(−)	(−)	(−)
Subclinical TB non-infectious	(+)	(−)	(−)
Subclinical TB infectious	(+)	(+)	(−)
Clinical TB non-infectious	(+)	(−)	(+)
Clinical TB infectious	(+)	(+)	(+)
Outcomes			
Self-cleared	(−) or (+)	(−)	(−) or (+) but never treated for TB
Infected	(+)	(−)	(−) but remains at risk
Full recovery	(+) residual	(−)	(−) and no post-TB functional impairment
Post-TB	(++)	(+)	(−) or (+) with functional disability due to TB pathology damage
Death	(+++)	(+) or (++)	(+++)

Table 1.
TB disease dimensions and outcomes.

are often characterised by the obstructive lobular pneumonia [81]. The 'tree-in-bud' sign on X-ray and CT images indicates inflammatory changes in the bronchioles, which typically resolve after a few months of treatment. If left untreated, pneumonia may either regress or progress into caseous pneumonia.

Upon treatment initiation, the conversion of sputum cultures from positive to negative serves as the key indicator for the commencement of the bacilli eradication process and the interruption of transmission. While the stochastic 2-week rule of isolation post-treatment initiation, considered a proxy for culture-to-negative conversion, has not been confirmed in systematic reviews [82], the combination of the decrease in viable bacilli burden, reduced frequency of cough, and improved clinical presentation are all considered when determining infection control measures. TB treatment duration may last from 4 months for non-severe drug susceptible smear-negative childhood TB [83] up to 24 months or longer for extensively drug-resistant (XDR) TB. In the latter, the burden of treatment-related side effects often equals the burden of the disease itself, leading to permanent organ damages not necessarily the ones with TB changes. Newly approved TB drugs and all-oral regimens significantly shortened treatment timelines and their burden [84]. However, increased use of these new drugs may result in drug resistance development to these therapeutics.

Permanent lung pathology often follows treatment for pulmonary TB. Post-tuberculosis lung disease (PTLD) often includes permanent lung changes, such as cavities, bronchiectasis, and fibrosis [85]. Clinically, these changes may manifest as a chronic respiratory disease with abnormalities in spirometry, reduced vital lung capacity, decreased exercise tolerance, and increased susceptibility to reinfection including TB recurrence [86]. The patient's quality of life is often affected [87]. Follow-up care involves pulmonary rehabilitation, vaccinations, and smoking cessation programmes [88].

6. Local tissue destruction in extrapulmonary TB

Extrapulmonary TB develops when *Mtb* spreads hematogenously to various organs beyond the lungs. It occurs either from infected lymph nodes or through local tissue

Type	Pathology and clinical presentation	Reference
TB lymphadenitis	Pathology: soft caseous mass replacing lymphatic tissue with presence of numerous acid-fast bacilli. Symptoms: progressively enlarging lymph nodes with contiguous spread to surrounding tissues forming appearance of so-called scrofula in the neck region; visually distinct and palpable mass may not be associated with fever or cachexia.	[89, 90]
TB meningitis	Pathology: usually paucibacillary inflammation of meninges; possible tuberculous granulomas [Rich foci] spreading to sub-arachnoid space. Symptoms: increased intracranial pressure with fever, headache, and vomiting; Complications: hydrocephalus, cranial nerve palsies, perforating vasculitis leading to hemi- or quadriplegia.	[91]
TB pericarditis	Pathology: purulent pericardial effusion with fibrin strands and high level of adenosine deaminase. Symptoms: progressive fatigue and dyspnoea with fever, distended neck veins and muffled heart sounds; constrictive pericarditis leading to heart tamponade.	[92]
Laryngeal TB	Pathology: usually evolution of the pulmonary disease and rarely confined to the larynx only granulomatous infiltration, which may be associated with caseous necrosis in the histopathology. Symptoms: hoarseness of the voice or its loss and pain are most frequent symptoms, often initially attributed to malignancy.	[93, 94]
Intestinal TB	Pathology: Transmural necrotising granulomatous inflammation. Symptoms: abdominal pain, risk of intestinal perforation and peritonitis, fistulation to other organs, "acute" abdomen, sepsis.	[95]
TB peritonitis	Symptoms: abdominal distension, pain, and fever; ascitic fluid with high protein and adenosine deaminase content; multiple enlarged mesenteric nodes, thickened peritoneum with presence of miliary nodules (tubercles).	[96]
Urogenital TB	Pathology: invasion of renal parenchyma, haematogenic foci, renal lesions evolving into renal abscesses; involvement of ureter and bladder through lymphatic system. Symptoms: Haematuria, dysuria or sterile pyuria, unilateral obstruction more frequently progressing to local complications of ureter stenosis and renal failure; urological or gynaecological complications in form of oligospermia and vaginal bleeding respectively.	[97, 98]
Splenic TB	Pathology: Necrotic nodules throughout splenic parenchyma with or without purulent discharge; granulomatous inflammation with caseous necrosis. Symptoms: abdominal pain on the left side, splenomegaly.	[99]
Spinal TB	Pathology: destruction of usually thoracic vertebrae with kyphotic deformation of spine and local lymphadenopathy. Symptoms: spinal cord compression symptoms with various levels of neurological symptoms, pain.	[100]
Ocular TB	Pathology: intra-ocular inflammation of uvea and retina (uveitis/retinitis); choroidal granulomas, keratic precipitates, retinal vasculitis. Symptoms: deterioration in vision, systemic symptoms; Complications: optic neuropathy and sight loss.	[101, 102]

Table 2.
Presentation in extrapulmonary tuberculosis.

destruction, allowing bacilli to enter capillaries and then the bloodstream to infect distant sites. In some cases, physiologically drained alveolar fluid containing infected cells can pass to the pharyngeal cavity, and if not destroyed by gastric acid, *Mtb* can travel to the intestines, causing intestinal TB. Interestingly, studies indicate no significant differences in the cellular composition of granulomas between different organ sites [43], confirming it is a pathogen-reactive process. Examples of the extra-pulmonary TB presentation are summarised in **Table 2**.

7. *Mtb* antigens in diagnosis: From microscopy and sputum culture to DNA-based assays

Tuberculin, a heat-killed culture filtrate of *Mtb* antigens, has been used in diagnostics as a tuberculin skin test (TST) since its development by Koch in 1890. Purified protein derivative (PPD) is a refined version of the original tuberculin, significantly reduced in polysaccharides, nucleic acids and lipid content that was likely responsible for adverse reactions to early forms [103]. PPD is enriched in members of the *Esx* family, with *GroEl, GroEs, DnaK* and *HspX* contributing up to 60% of its content [104]. TST test involves subcutaneous injection of PPD and measurement of the induration at the injection site after 48–72 hours. Alternatively, interferon-gamma release assays (IGRAs) tests measure the immune responses by detecting IFN-γ secretion from activated T cells in response to TB-specific antigens. Both TST and IGRA can be used to test for TB infection; however, TST shows lower specificity in individuals with recent Bacillus Calmette-Guerin (BCG) vaccination or immunosuppression. According to the WHO, neither test should be preferred over the other for predicting progression to active TB disease [105], with the choice of the test typically guided by TST stock availability and access to an adequately equipped laboratory. IGRA tests do not provide added benefit over conventional microbiological methods in diagnosing active TB.

In laboratory TB diagnostics, bright-field microscopy with Ziehl-Neelsen staining and fluorescence microscopy with Auramine-O are two major microscopy techniques. Both staining techniques rely on the high lipid content of the mycobacterial cell wall, which retains the stain. Automated image processing methods can help with the identification of bacilli in these stains [106]. Most rapid diagnostic tests rely on *Mtb* DNA detection, and these methods have been consolidated in the WHO module 3 guidelines on TB in 2024 [105]. One notable exception to nucleic acid-based tests is the lateral flow urine lipoarabinomannan (LAM) assay. The LAM assay detects glycolipid lipoarabinomannan, a component of mycobacterial cell wall, in urine samples. It is particularly suitable for diagnosing TB in individuals co-infected with HIV [107, 108], despite its overall lower sensitivity and specificity compared to DNA-based tests.

The TB diagnostic pipeline has expanded significantly to include targeted next-generation sequencing with the aim for culture-free whole genome sequencing [WGS] directly from complex samples as a rapid response to TB outbreak tracking, TB surveillance, and the control of resistance to anti-tuberculosis drugs [109]. Currently, as a nationwide strategy, WGS is predominantly deployed in high-resource, low-burden countries [110] and is typically performed only on *Mtb* after it has been grown and isolated in culture. Pan-susceptibility testing is limited to first-line anti-tuberculosis drugs [111]. Despite progress in cost reduction, as of 2024, the cost of a single clinical application remains around 10x higher than PCR-based rapid diagnostic tests, making it inaccessible for widespread implementation in

Drug	Genetic and inhibition factors	Reference
Rifampicin	rpoA, **rpoB**, rpoC (RNA polymerase) Rv2752c (ribonuclease)	[117, 118]
Isoniazid	**katG** (catalase peroxidase), Rv2752c, tap (multidrug efflux transport protein) **inhA** (NADH-dependent enoyl-[acyl-carrier-protein] reductase) mshA ndh (membrane NADH dehydrogenase), **ahpC** (alkyl hydroperoxide reductase C) fadE24 (acyl-CoA dehydrogenase), **fabG1** (fatty acid biosynthesis pathway, first reduction step)	[119]
Ethambutol	embA, **embB**, embC, embR (family of arabinosyltransferases), ubiA (Decaprenylphosphoryl-5-phosphoribose synthase)	[120, 121]
Pyrazinamide	**pncA** (pyrazinamidase/nicotinamidase) rpsA (ribosomal protein) panD (aspartate 1-decarboxylase precursor) clpC1 (clp protease—degradation of misfolded proteins) PPE35, tap kefB (membrane transport protein)	[122, 123]
Moxifloxacin (and other fluoroquinolones)	**gyrA**, **gyrB** (DNA gyrase and topoisomerase)	[124, 125]
Bedaquiline	atpE (ATP synthase), mmpR, pepQ, Rv0678 (protein regulator of mmpS5-mmpL5 efflux pump)	[126–128]
Clofazimine	mmpR (transcriptional regulatory protein) Rv1979c (amino acid membrane transporter) pepQ (cytoplasmic peptidase), Rv0678	[126]
Linezolid	rplC, rrl—both ribosomal proteins	[126, 129]
Delamanid	ddn, fbiA, fbiC, fgd1—all associated with co-factor F_{420} structure or functions	[130]
Pretomanid	ddn (deazaflavin-dependent nitroreductase), fgd1, fbiA-C	[131, 132]
Cycloserine	iniA (isoniazid-inducible protein) alr (alanine racemase) ddl (D-alanine-D-alanine ligase) ald (alanine dehydrogenase) cycA (D-serine/alanine/glycine transporter protein)	[133, 134]
Amikacin, Kanamycin	**Rrs** (ribosomal protein) **eis** (GCN5-related N-acetyltransferase) whiB7 (transcriptional regulatory protein, thyA (thymidylate synthase)	[135]
p-aminosalicylic acid	thyA, folC (dihydrofolate synthase) dfrA (dihydrofolate reductase) ribD (riboflavin biosynthesis)	[136, 137]
Ethionamide	ethA (FAD-containing monooxygenase) ethR (transcriptional regulatory protein) kasA (b-ketoacyl-acyl carrier protein (ACP) synthase), **inhA**	[138, 139]

Genes for which WHO-endorsed rapid diagnostic methods are available are highlighted in bold.

Table 3.
List of Mtb genes contributing to drug resistance in current therapies.

low-resource countries. However, in these settings, WGS could be particularly useful for tracking the emergence of new, highly virulent variants and variants resistant to new and established anti-TB drugs [112]. Markers of resistance and targeting in therapeutic regimens: overview.

TB treatment, due to its complexity and long duration, is linked to the risk of drug resistance development. In 2019, approximately 5% (half a million) of 10 million people diagnosed with TB developed resistance to rifampicin (RR-TB), and 10% developed isoniazid-resistant TB [113] remaining susceptible to rifampicin. The introduction of DNA-based rapid diagnostic tools has significantly improved the detection of rifampicin resistance, with 73% of bacteriologically confirmed TB patients being tested for rifampicin resistance in 2022 [1]. There has been marked improvement in diagnostics of resistance to other first-line drugs and gradual progress in identifying resistance to second- and third-line therapies.

In 2021, WHO developed a comprehensive atlas of *Mtb* genomic mutations [113]. The table below summarises key *Mtb* genes that contribute to drug resistance, with those genes for which WHO-endorsed rapid methods are available highlighted in **bold** [114, 115]. Rapid diagnostics are not yet available for bedaquiline, linezolid, delamanid, and pretomanid [116], for which next-generation sequencing is considered a viable alternative (**Table 3**).

8. TB vaccine - From BCG to subunit vaccines: Target antigens

Vaccination with a live attenuated strain of *Mycobacterium bovis*, the Bacillus Calmette-Guerin (BCG), remains the cornerstone vaccine against TB since its first use in 1919, despite its limitations in stimulating long-term protective immune responses in adults. Due to the wealth of existing safety data on BCG, methodology, and established production systems, it provides a benchmark for new vaccine candidates, which must demonstrate not only non-inferiority but also clear superiority to BCG to advance in clinical trials. BCG does not prevent TB infection but rather increases resistance to disease progression by inhibiting uncontrollable *Mtb* multiplication and its dissemination. This is achieved by promoting the recruitment of activated lymphocytes, reducing granuloma size, and minimising necrosis. BCG attenuation is linked to the deletion of the RD1 region, which includes the protein secretion system Esx-1. It is further supplemented by tandem duplications of genes required to grow on glycerol and downregulation of genes associated with fatty acid degradation [140]. However, the changes in lipid composition have to be finely balanced to avoid compromising vaccine effectiveness [141].

Other whole mycobacteria vaccines tested against TB, included *Mycobacterium obuense* SRL-DAR-01 [142, 143], and Immuvac (MIP)—heat-killed *Mycobacterium indicus* pranii, which were predominantly tested as immune boosters [144]. Other poly-antigenic compositions include RUTI, which consists of detoxified wall fragments of Mtb bacilli grown under stressful conditions [145, 146].

Last quarter century, the field of subunit vaccines has been developing in line with advancements in genomics and protein expression techniques. New research methods in analytical technology, such as immunoproteomics and immunopeptidomics, supplemented by bioinformatic approaches, aim to identify the antigens presented by infected cells to identify the ones that sensitised immune cells respond to the most [147, 148]. The purpose of these mass spectrometry-based tools is to deliver experimental proof for the design of new subunit vaccines. However, despite the *Mycobacterium tuberculosis* genome consisting of over 4000 open reading frames (ORFs), only 18 antigen candidates are currently tested in clinical trials [149]. These include Ag85A, Ag85b, the **ESAT6-CFP10** complex, **TB10.4**, PPE18 **(Mtb39a),** PPE42, **PPE68,** PepA **(Mtb32a),** EspA, EspC, **espI, esxV, esxW, Rv1813c, MPT64, MPT70, MPT83, and Rv2660c,** with those not expressed in an ortholog form in BCG marked in bold.

New forefronts are explored by the first mRNA vaccine, BNT164, which qualified for dose-finding Phase 1 studies as BNT164a1 and BNT164b1 [150]. The antigenic composition of these vaccines is currently undisclosed. In view of the lack of established correlates of protection, these vaccines represent not only methodological innovation but also the results of their testing will verify whether mRNA vaccines can induce strong and comprehensive immune responses against TB.

As of 2023, there are 16 TB vaccine candidates in testing [1], with one candidate vaccine, M72/$AS01_E$, meeting WHO's preferred product characteristics [151]. While the other candidates progressed through the testing pipeline ([152, 153]), a completely new subunit vaccine candidate, H107e/CAF1-b, entered phase 1 testing. It includes 8 antigens with ESAT-6 in four repeats, marking the highest number of simultaneously co-expressed antigens for the subunit vaccine in TB vaccinology. It was specifically designed to express antigens absent or nearly absent in BCG in order to enhance its immunogenicity in the BCG-prime and H107e/CAF1-b booster vaccination strategy. This objective was achieved in the preclinical model [154], where protective and synergistic responses were recorded at 20 weeks post-simultaneous vaccination of BCG and H107e/CAF1-b, but, notably, not at the early time point of 4 weeks. There was a significant increase in IL-17 and IFN-γ cytokines. In October 2023, Phase 1a, dose-finding, followed by Phase 1b, double-blind, randomised, placebo-controlled trials were initiated in South Africa with the outcomes expected in 2026 [155].

9. Summary

Mycobacterium tuberculosis co-evolved with humans for at least 100,000 years, possibly even pre-dating the emergence of *Homo sapiens* [137]. During this long evolutionary period, the pathogen has developed a highly effective lifecycle, characterised by a long latency phase and the ability to initiate infection with a single or a few bacilli. This strategy has proven successful, with 20% of the global human population currently latently infected. High mycolic acids and lipids content, many of them unique for mycobacteria, pose difficulty for effective antigen presentation. At the same time, immunodominance of small proteinaceous antigens and key *Mtb* virulence factors leads to overstimulation and exhaustion of cell-mediated immunity before the generation of long-term memory cells takes place. TB's clinical picture is one of slow tissue destruction, as much by inflammation as the pathogen. The significant progress in new therapeutics against TB has yet to be matched by the advancement in TB vaccinology. Equally, the DNA-based rapid diagnostic tools are likely to become a driver of the clinical management personalisation in TB as long as their development and accessibility extend beyond first-line therapy drugs. Targeted immunotherapy has recorded modest success so far, with broadly acting steroids widely accepted in the clinical management of TB meningitis but less uniformly across other TB presentations. Host-directed repurposed drugs like metformin and vitamin D are effective in certain susceptible patients' subpopulations. The current practice of polypharmacotherapy in TB poses a barrier to adding more drugs of supporting roles, which may change with newer, all-oral regimens. The results of a recent trial investigating the role of improved nutrition in household contacts of patients with microbiologically confirmed pulmonary TB showed a significant reduction in TB incidence [156], and, less distinctly, other studies indicated better treatment outcomes in the population of TB patients [157]—this approach may present a socially acceptable strategy that exercises pleiotropic effects on multiple immune pathways to result in improved treatment outcomes. Mtb remains one of the most successful infectious pathogens, where only concerted long-term efforts by all stakeholders in public health, diagnostics, pharmacotherapy, and vaccinology will be able to change the overall picture and bring the disease under control.

Acknowledgements

The author would like to acknowledge Dr. Charles J Woodrow, Consultant in Infectious Diseases at Oxford University Hospital NHS Trust, Oxford, United Kingdom, for his input.

Author details

Karolina D. Witt[1,2]

1 University of Oxford, Oxford, United Kingdom

2 John Warin Infectious Diseases Ward, Oxford University Hospitals NHS Foundation Trust, Oxford, United Kingdom

*Address all correspondence to: karolina.witt@ouh.nhs.uk

References

[1] WHO. Global tuberculosis report 2023. Available from: https://www.who.int/publications/i/item/9789240083851 [Accessed: 24 July 2024]

[2] Pinto PFPS et al. Incidence and risk factors of tuberculosis among 420 854 household contacts of patients with tuberculosis in the 100 million Brazilian cohort (2004-18): A cohort study. The Lancet Infectious Diseases. 2024;**24**(1):46-56. DOI: 10.1016/S1473-3099(23)00371-7

[3] Barriers to access—TB AlertTB Alert. Available from: https://www.tbalert.org/about-tb/global-tb-challenges/barriers-to-accessing-treatment/ [Accessed: 3 December 2024]

[4] Rosales-Klintz S et al. Guidance for programmatic management of latent tuberculosis infection in the European Union/European economic area. The European Respiratory Journal. 2019;**53**(1). DOI: 10.1183/13993003.02077-2018

[5] Demay C et al. SITVITWEB—A publicly available international multimarker database for studying *Mycobacterium tuberculosis* genetic diversity and molecular epidemiology. Infection, Genetics and Evolution. 2012;**12**(4):755-766. DOI: 10.1016/J.MEEGID.2012.02.004

[6] Comas I et al. Out-of-Africa migration and Neolithic coexpansion of *Mycobacterium tuberculosis* with modern humans. Nature Genetics. 2013;**45**(10):1176-1182. DOI: 10.1038/NG.2744

[7] Torrelles JB, Schlesinger LS. Integrating lung physiology, immunology, and tuberculosis. Trends in Microbiology. 2017;**25**(8):688-697. DOI: 10.1016/j.tim.2017.03.007

[8] Donald PR, Diacon AH, Thee S. Anton Ghon and his colleagues and their studies of the primary focus and complex of tuberculosis infection and their relevance for the twenty-first century. Respiration. 2021;**100**(7):557-567. DOI: 10.1159/000509522

[9] Levitte S, Adams KN, Berg RD, Cosma CL, Urdahl KB, Ramakrishnan L. Mycobacterial acid tolerance enables phagolysosomal survival and establishment of tuberculous infection in vivo. Cell Host & Microbe. 2016;**20**(2):250-258. DOI: 10.1016/J.CHOM.2016.07.007

[10] Vázquez CL et al. Experimental selection of long-term intracellular mycobacteria. Cellular Microbiology. 2014;**16**(9):1425-1440. DOI: 10.1111/CMI.12303

[11] Mokrousov I et al. Insight into pathogenomics and phylogeography of hypervirulent and highly-lethal *Mycobacterium tuberculosis* strain cluster. BMC Infectious Diseases. 2023;**23**(1). DOI: 10.1186/S12879-023-08413-7

[12] Singh SK et al. HIV interferes with *Mycobacterium tuberculosis* antigen presentation in human dendritic cells. The American Journal of Pathology. 2016;**186**(12):3083-3093. DOI: 10.1016/J.AJPATH.2016.08.003

[13] Van Crevel R, Ottenhoff THM, Van der Meer JWM. Innate immunity to *Mycobacterium tuberculosis*. Clinical Microbiology Reviews. 2002;**15**(2):294-309. DOI: 10.1128/CMR.15.2.294-309.2002

[14] Hossain MM, Norazmi MN. Pattern recognition receptors and cytokines in *Mycobacterium tuberculosis* infection—The double-edged sword? BioMed Research International. 2013;**2013**. DOI: 10.1155/2013/179174

[15] Cambier CJ, Falkow S, Ramakrishnan L. Host evasion and exploitation schemes of *Mycobacterium tuberculosis*. Cell. 2014;**159**(7):1497-1509. DOI: 10.1016/J.CELL.2014.11.024

[16] Wong D, Bach H, Sun J, Hmama Z, Av-Gay Y. *Mycobacterium tuberculosis* protein tyrosine phosphatase (PtpA) excludes host vacuolar-H+-ATPase to inhibit phagosome acidification. Proceedings of the National Academy of Sciences of the United States of America. 2011;**108**(48):19371-19376. DOI: 10.1073/PNAS.1109201108

[17] Vergne I, Chua J, Singh SB, Deretic V. Cell biology of *Mycobacterium tuberculosis* phagosome. Annual Review of Cell and Developmental Biology. 2004;**20**:367-394. DOI: 10.1146/ANNUREV.CELLBIO.20.010403.114015

[18] Pradhan G, Shrivastva R, Mukhopadhyay S. Mycobacterial PknG targets the Rab7l1 signaling pathway to inhibit phagosome-lysosome fusion. Journal of Immunology. 2018;**201**(5):1421-1433. DOI: 10.4049/JIMMUNOL.1800530

[19] Serafini A et al. *Mycobacterium tuberculosis* requires glyoxylate shunt and reverse methylcitrate cycle for lactate and pyruvate metabolism. Molecular Microbiology. 2019;**112**(4):1284. DOI: 10.1111/MMI.14362

[20] Karamooz E, Harriff MJ, Narayanan GA, Worley A, Lewinsohn DM. MR1 recycling and blockade of endosomal trafficking reveal distinguishable antigen presentation pathways between *Mycobacterium tuberculosis* infection and exogenously delivered antigens. Scientific Reports. 2019;**9**(1). DOI: 10.1038/S41598-019-41402-Y

[21] Leddy O, White FM, Bryson BD. Immunopeptidomics reveals determinants of *Mycobacterium tuberculosis* antigen presentation on MHC class I. eLife. 2023;**12**. DOI: 10.7554/ELIFE.84070

[22] Vordermeier HM et al. Conserved immune recognition hierarchy of mycobacterial PE/PPE proteins during infection in natural hosts. PLoS One. 2012;**7**(8). DOI: 10.1371/JOURNAL.PONE.0040890

[23] Behr MA, Edelstein PH, Ramakrishnan L. Revisiting the timetable of tuberculosis. The BMJ. 2018;**362**. DOI: 10.1136/BMJ.K2738

[24] Pal R, Bisht MK, Mukhopadhyay S. Secretory proteins of *Mycobacterium tuberculosis* and their roles in modulation of host immune responses: Focus on therapeutic targets. The FEBS Journal. 2022;**289**(14):4146-4171. DOI: 10.1111/FEBS.16369

[25] Portal-Celhay C et al. *Mycobacterium tuberculosis* EsxH inhibits ESCRT-dependent CD4+ T-cell activation. Nature Microbiology. 2016;**2**. DOI: 10.1038/NMICROBIOL.2016.232

[26] Gehring AJ, Dobos KM, Belisle JT, Harding CV, Boom WH. *Mycobacterium tuberculosis* LprG (Rv1411c): A novel TLR-2 ligand that inhibits human macrophage class II MHC antigen processing. Journal of Immunology. 2004;**173**(4):2660-2668. DOI: 10.4049/JIMMUNOL.173.4.2660

[27] Bhat KH, Srivastava S, Kotturu SK, Ghosh S, Mukhopadhyay S. The PPE2

protein of *Mycobacterium tuberculosis* translocates to host nucleus and inhibits nitric oxide production. Scientific Reports. 2017;7. DOI: 10.1038/SREP39706

[28] Bhat KH, Ahmed A, Kumar S, Sharma P, Mukhopadhyay S. Role of PPE18 protein in intracellular survival and pathogenicity of *Mycobacterium tuberculosis* in mice. PLoS One. 2012;7(12). DOI: 10.1371/JOURNAL.PONE.0052601

[29] Samuel LP et al. Expression, production and release of the Eis protein by *Mycobacterium tuberculosis* during infection of macrophages and its effect on cytokine secretion. Microbiology (Reading). 2007;**153**(Pt 2):529-540. DOI: 10.1099/MIC.0.2006/002642-0

[30] Yaseen I, Kaur P, Nandicoori VK, Khosla S. Mycobacteria modulate host epigenetic machinery by Rv1988 methylation of a non-tail arginine of histone H3. Nature Communications. 2015;**6**. DOI: 10.1038/NCOMMS9922

[31] Köster S et al. *Mycobacterium tuberculosis* is protected from NADPH oxidase and LC3-associated phagocytosis by the LCP protein CpsA. Proceedings of the National Academy of Sciences of the United States of America. 2017;**114**(41):E8711-E8720. DOI: 10.1073/PNAS.1707792114

[32] Lopes RL, Borges TJ, Zanin RF, Bonorino C. IL-10 is required for polarization of macrophages to M2-like phenotype by mycobacterial DnaK (heat shock protein 70). Cytokine. 2016;**85**:123-129. DOI: 10.1016/J.CYTO.2016.06.018

[33] Cambier CJ, O'Leary SM, O'Sullivan MP, Keane J, Ramakrishnan L. Phenolic glycolipid facilitates mycobacterial escape from microbicidal tissue-resident macrophages. Immunity. 2017;**47**(3):552-565.e4. DOI: 10.1016/J.IMMUNI.2017.08.003

[34] Divangahi M et al. *Mycobacterium tuberculosis* evades macrophage defenses by inhibiting plasma membrane repair. Nature Immunology. 2009;**10**(8):899-906. DOI: 10.1038/NI.1758

[35] Behar SM, Divangahi M, Remold HG. Evasion of innate immunity by *Mycobacterium tuberculosis*: Is death an exit strategy? Nature Reviews. Microbiology. 2010;**8**(9):668-674. DOI: 10.1038/NRMICRO2387

[36] Amaral EP et al. A major role for ferroptosis in *Mycobacterium tuberculosis*-induced cell death and tissue necrosis. The Journal of Experimental Medicine. 2019;**216**(3):556-570. DOI: 10.1084/JEM.20181776

[37] Olson GS et al. Type I interferon decreases macrophage energy metabolism during mycobacterial infection. Cell Reports. 2021;**35**(9). DOI: 10.1016/J.CELREP.2021.109195

[38] Ottenhoff THM et al. Genome-wide expression profiling identifies type 1 interferon response pathways in active tuberculosis. PLoS One. 2012;7(9). DOI: 10.1371/JOURNAL.PONE.0045839

[39] Feng Y et al. Platelets direct monocyte differentiation into epithelioid-like multinucleated giant foam cells with suppressive capacity upon mycobacterial stimulation. The Journal of Infectious Diseases. 2014;**210**(11):1700-1710. DOI: 10.1093/INFDIS/JIU355

[40] Lerner TR et al. Lymphatic endothelial cells are a replicative niche for *Mycobacterium tuberculosis*. The Journal of Clinical Investigation. 2016;**126**(3):1093-1108. DOI: 10.1172/JCI83379

[41] Ardain A et al. Group 3 innate lymphoid cells mediate early protective immunity against tuberculosis. Nature. 2019;**570**(7762):528-532. DOI: 10.1038/S41586-019-1276-2

[42] Magcwebeba T, Dorhoi A, Du Plessis N. The emerging role of myeloid-derived suppressor cells in tuberculosis. Frontiers in Immunology. 2019;**10**(APR). DOI: 10.3389/FIMMU.2019.00917

[43] McCaffrey EF et al. The immunoregulatory landscape of human tuberculosis granulomas. Nature Immunology. 2022;**23**(2):318. DOI: 10.1038/S41590-021-01121-X

[44] Choreño Parra JA, Martínez Zúñiga N, Jiménez Zamudio LA, Jiménez Álvarez LA, Salinas Lara C, Zúñiga J. Memory of natural killer cells: A new chance against *Mycobacterium tuberculosis*? Frontiers in Immunology. 2017;**8**(AUG). DOI: 10.3389/FIMMU.2017.00967

[45] Moorlag SJCFM et al. BCG vaccination induces long-term functional reprogramming of human neutrophils. Cell Reports. 2020;**33**(7):108387. DOI: 10.1016/J.CELREP.2020.108387

[46] Srivastava S, Grace PS, Ernst JD. Antigen export reduces antigen presentation and limits T cell control of *M. tuberculosis*. Cell Host & Microbe. 2016;**19**(1):44-54. DOI: 10.1016/J.CHOM.2015.12.003

[47] Marakalala MJ et al. Inflammatory signaling in human tuberculosis granulomas is spatially organized. Nature Medicine. 2016;**22**(5):531-538. DOI: 10.1038/NM.4073

[48] Yamagami H et al. Trehalose 6,6'-dimycolate (cord factor) of *Mycobacterium tuberculosis* induces foreign-body- and hypersensitivity-type granulomas in mice. Infection and Immunity. 2001;**69**(2):810-815. DOI: 10.1128/IAI.69.2.810-815.2001

[49] Lewinsohn DA, Heinzel AS, Gardner JM, Zhu L, Alderson MR, LewinsohnDM.*Mycobacteriumtuberculosis*-specific CD8+ T cells preferentially recognize heavily infected cells. American Journal of Respiratory and Critical Care Medicine. 2003;**168**(11):1346-1352. DOI: 10.1164/RCCM.200306-837OC

[50] Sarathy JP, Dartois V. Caseum: A niche for *Mycobacterium tuberculosis* drug-tolerant persisters. Clinical Microbiology Reviews. 2020;**33**(3). DOI: 10.1128/CMR.00159-19

[51] Mitchison DA. The search for new sterilizing anti-tuberculosis drugs. Frontiers in Bioscience. 2004;**9**:1059-1072. DOI: 10.2741/1293

[52] Hunter RL, Venkataprasad N, Olsen MR. The role of trehalose dimycolate (cord factor) on morphology of virulent *M. tuberculosis* in vitro. Tuberculosis. 2006;**86**(5):349-356. DOI: 10.1016/j.tube.2005.08.017

[53] Li S et al. Elevated natural killer cell-mediated cytotoxicity is associated with cavity formation in pulmonary tuberculosis patients. Journal of Immunology Research. 2021;**2021**. DOI: 10.1155/2021/7925903

[54] Nyendak MR et al. *Mycobacterium tuberculosis* specific CD8(+) T cells rapidly decline with antituberculosis treatment. PLoS One. 2013;**8**(12). DOI: 10.1371/JOURNAL.PONE.0081564

[55] Fletcher HA. Systems approaches to correlates of protection and progression to TB disease. Seminars in Immunology. 2018;**39**:81-87. DOI: 10.1016/j.smim.2018.10.001

[56] Balamurugan A, Sharma SK, Mehra NK. Human leukocyte antigen class I supertypes influence susceptibility and severity of tuberculosis. The Journal of Infectious Diseases. 2004;**189**(5):805-811. DOI: 10.1086/381689

[57] Sveinbjornsson G et al. HLA class II sequence variants influence tuberculosis risk in populations of European ancestry. Nature Genetics. 2016;**48**(3):318-322. DOI: 10.1038/NG.3498

[58] Thye T et al. IL10 haplotype associated with tuberculin skin test response but not with pulmonary TB. PLoS One. 2009;**4**(5). DOI: 10.1371/JOURNAL.PONE.0005420

[59] Boussiotis VA et al. IL-10-producing T cells suppress immune responses in anergic tuberculosis patients. Journal of Clinical Investigation. 2000;**105**(9):1317-1325. DOI: 10.1172/JCI9918

[60] Böhme J et al. Metformin enhances anti-mycobacterial responses by educating CD8+ T-cell immunometabolic circuits. Nature Communications. 2020;**11**(1). DOI: 10.1038/S41467-020-19095-Z

[61] Frazier-Mironer A et al. Adverse effects of biologics: A network meta-analysis and cochrane overview. Cochrane Database of Systematic Reviews. 2011;**2011**(2):483-490. DOI: 10.1002/14651858.CD008794.PUB2

[62] Sartori NS, Picon P, Papke A, Neyeloff JL, da Silva Chakr RM. A population-based study of tuberculosis incidence among rheumatic disease patients under anti-TNF treatment. PLoS One. 2019;**14**(12). DOI: 10.1371/JOURNAL.PONE.0224963

[63] Harari A et al. Dominant TNF-α+ *Mycobacterium tuberculosis*-specific CD4+ T cell responses discriminate between latent infection and active disease. Nature Medicine. 2011;**17**(3):372-377. DOI: 10.1038/NM.2299

[64] Luo Y et al. Activation phenotype of *Mycobacterium tuberculosis*-specific CD4+ T cells promoting the discrimination between active tuberculosis and latent tuberculosis infection. Frontiers in Immunology. 2021;**12**. DOI: 10.3389/FIMMU.2021.721013

[65] Rozot V et al. *Mycobacterium tuberculosis*-specific CD8+ T cells are functionally and phenotypically different between latent infection and active disease. European Journal of Immunology. 2013;**43**(6):1568-1577. DOI: 10.1002/EJI.201243262

[66] Coppola M et al. Cell-mediated immune responses to in vivo-expressed and stage-specific *Mycobacterium tuberculosis* antigens in latent and active tuberculosis across different age groups. Frontiers in Immunology. 2020;**11**. DOI: 10.3389/FIMMU.2020.00103

[67] Andersson J, Samarina A, Fink J, Rahman S, Grundström S. Impaired expression of perforin and granulysin in CD8+ T cells at the site of infection in human chronic pulmonary tuberculosis. Infection and Immunity. 2007;**75**(11):5210. DOI: 10.1128/IAI.00624-07

[68] Witt KD. Role of MHC class I pathways in *Mycobacterium tuberculosis* antigen presentation. Frontiers in Cellular and Infection Microbiology. 2023;**13**. DOI: 10.3389/FCIMB.2023.1107884

[69] Lopez K et al. CD1b tetramers broadly detect T cells that correlate with mycobacterial exposure but not tuberculosis disease state. Frontiers in Immunology. 2020;**11**. DOI: 10.3389/FIMMU.2020.00199

[70] Harriff MJ et al. MR1 displays the microbial metabolome driving selective MR1-restricted T cell receptor usage. Science Immunology. 2018;**3**(25). DOI: 10.1126/SCIIMMUNOL.AAO2556

[71] WHO. Tuberculosis. Available from: https://www.who.int/health-topics/tuberculosis#tab=tab_1 [Accessed: 19 August 2024]

[72] Sossen B et al. The natural history of untreated pulmonary tuberculosis in adults: A systematic review and meta-analysis. The Lancet Respiratory Medicine. 2023;**11**(4):367-379. DOI: 10.1016/S2213-2600(23)00097-8

[73] Horton KC, Richards AS, Emery JC, Esmail H, Houben RMGJ. Reevaluating progression and pathways following *Mycobacterium tuberculosis* infection within the spectrum of tuberculosis. Proceedings of the National Academy of Sciences of the United States of America. 2023;**120**(47). DOI: 10.1073/PNAS.2221186120

[74] Lambert ML, Hasker E, Van Deun A, Roberfroid D, Boelaert M, Van der Stuyft P. Recurrence in tuberculosis: Relapse or reinfection? Lancet Infectious Diseases. 2003;**3**(5):282-287. DOI: 10.1016/S1473-3099(03)00607-8

[75] Patterson B, Wood R. Is cough really necessary for TB transmission? Tuberculosis (Edinburgh, Scotland). 2019;**117**:31. DOI: 10.1016/J.TUBE.2019.05.003

[76] Seddon JA, McQuaid CF, Mafirakureva N, Hesseling AC, Fox GJ, Dodd PJ. Household contact management and preventive treatment for drug-resistant tuberculosis. The Lancet Global Health. 2024;**12**(9):e1387-e1388. DOI: 10.1016/S2214-109X(24)00265-1

[77] Cohen A, Mathiasen VD, Schön T, Wejse C. The global prevalence of latent tuberculosis: A systematic review and meta-analysis. The European Respiratory Journal. 2019;**54**(3). DOI: 10.1183/13993003.00655-2019

[78] Marx FM, Hauer B, Menzies NA, Haas W, Perumal N. Targeting screening and treatment for latent tuberculosis infection towards asylum seekers from high-incidence countries—A model-based cost-effectiveness analysis. BMC Public Health. 2021;**21**(1):2172. DOI: 10.1186/S12889-021-12142-4

[79] Long A et al. The technology behind TB DEPOT: A novel public analytics platform integrating tuberculosis clinical, genomic, and radiological data for visual and statistical exploration. Journal of the American Medical Informatics Association. 2020;**28**(1):71. DOI: 10.1093/JAMIA/OCAA228

[80] Coussens AK et al. International consensus classification of early tuberculosis states to guide research for improved care and prevention: A Delphi exercise. The Lancet Respiratory Medicine. 2024;**12**(6):484. DOI: 10.1016/S2213-2600(24)00028-6

[81] Hunter RL. The pathogenesis of tuberculosis: The early infiltrate of post-primary (adult pulmonary) tuberculosis: A distinct disease entity. Frontiers in Immunology. 2018;**9**(SEP). DOI: 10.3389/FIMMU.2018.02108

[82] Calderwood CJ et al. Dynamics of sputum conversion during effective tuberculosis treatment: A systematic review and meta-analysis. PLoS Medicine. 2021;**18**(4). DOI: 10.1371/JOURNAL.PMED.1003566

[83] Turkova A et al. Shorter treatment for nonsevere tuberculosis in African and Indian children. New England Journal of Medicine. 2022;**386**(10):911-922. DOI: 10.1056/NEJMOA2104535/

SUPPL_FILE/NEJMOA2104535_DATA-SHARING.PDF

[84] WHO. WHO consolidated guidelines on tuberculosis. Module 4: treatment - drug-resistant tuberculosis treatment, 2022 update | 15 December 2022: 133, 2022. Available from: https://www.who.int/publications/i/item/9789240063129 [Accessed: 6 October 2024]

[85] Meghji J, Simpson H, Squire SB, Mortimer K. A systematic review of the prevalence and pattern of imaging defined post-TB lung disease. PLoS One. 2016;**11**(8). DOI: 10.1371/JOURNAL.PONE.0161176

[86] Allwood BW, Byrne A, Meghji J, Rachow A, Van Der Zalm MM, Schoch OD. Post-tuberculosis lung disease: Clinical review of an under-recognised global challenge. Respiration. 2021;**100**(8):751-763. DOI: 10.1159/000512531

[87] Menzies NA et al. Lifetime burden of disease due to incident tuberculosis: A global reappraisal including post-tuberculosis sequelae. The Lancet Global Health. 2021;**9**(12):e1679-e1687. DOI: 10.1016/S2214-109X(21)00367-3

[88] Allwood BW et al. Post-tuberculosis lung health: Perspectives from the first international symposium. International Journal of Tuberculosis and Lung Disease. 2020;**24**(8):820-828. DOI: 10.5588/IJTLD.20.0067

[89] Miranti JP. Scrofula. Journal of the American College Health Association. 1968;**16**(4):409-410. DOI: 10.1056/NEJMICM050819/ASSET/E7146630-EA0C-4031-8646-2D722191A8BC/ASSETS/IMAGES/LARGE/NEJMICM050819_F1.JPG

[90] Ting K-C, Wang G-S. Paradoxical reaction in the treatment of scrofula. New England Journal of Medicine. 2020;**383**(18):1767-1767. DOI: 10.1056/NEJMICM2001912/ASSET/8D4B96B4-B0B6-4354-B243-D9869C59153F/ASSETS/IMAGES/LARGE/NEJMICM2001912_F1.JPG

[91] Donald PR, Schoeman JF. Tuberculous meningitis. New England Journal of Medicine. 2004;**351**(17):1719-1720. DOI: 10.1056/NEJMP048227

[92] Faria D, Freitas A, Fonseca HDF, Sacks CA. Tuberculous pericarditis. New England Journal of Medicine. 2018;**378**(20). DOI: 10.1056/NEJMICM1709552

[93] Agarwal R et al. Primary laryngeal tuberculosis: A series of 15 cases. Head and Neck Pathology. 2019;**13**(3):339. DOI: 10.1007/S12105-018-0970-Y

[94] Benwill JL, Sarria JC. Laryngeal tuberculosis in the United States of America: A forgotten disease. Scandinavian Journal of Infectious Diseases. 2014;**46**(4):241-249. DOI: 10.3109/00365548.2013.877157

[95] Oñate-Ocaña LF, Pérez-Díaz L. Intestinal tuberculosis. New England Journal of Medicine. 2022;**386**(13). DOI: 10.1056/NEJMICM2114345

[96] Okamoto K, Hatakeyama S, Sacks CA. Tuberculous peritonitis. New England Journal of Medicine. 2018;**379**(12). DOI: 10.1056/NEJMICM1713168

[97] Masuda H, Kamada K. Urinary tract tuberculosis. New England Journal of Medicine. 2016;**375**(11):1068-1068. DOI: 10.1056/NEJMICM1513715/ASSET/652FDB24-748C-4E8E-9E1E-F2214C5782D1/ASSETS/IMAGES/LARGE/NEJMICM1513715_F1.JPG

[98] Figueiredo AA, Lucon AM, Srougi M. Urogenital tuberculosis. Microbiol

Spectr. 2017;**5**(1). DOI: 10.1128/MICROBIOLSPEC.TNMI7-0015-2016

[99] Chen C-Y, Yang P-J, Sherman SV. Splenic tuberculosis. New England Journal of Medicine. 2023;**388**(4). DOI: 10.1056/NEJMICM2206174

[100] Jenks PJ, Stewart B. Vertebral tuberculosis. New England Journal of Medicine. 1998;**338**(23):1677-1677. DOI: 10.1056/NEJM199806043382306/ASSET/F0E96A11-87DC-43FE-9ADA-A3DE57B4DBB6/ASSETS/IMAGES/LARGE/NEJM199806043382306_F1.JPG

[101] Kon OM et al. BTS clinical statement for the diagnosis and management of ocular tuberculosis. BMJ Open Respiratory Research. 2022;**9**(1). DOI: 10.1136/BMJRESP-2022-001225

[102] Ezra DG, Pavesio CE. Chorioretinal granuloma in tuberculosis. New England Journal of Medicine. 2010;**363**(23):2248-2248. DOI: 10.1056/NEJMICM0912935/ASSET/FE4A137E-1ACE-49E8-AD54-43EB613BA880/ASSETS/IMAGES/LARGE/NEJMICM0912935_F1.JPG

[103] Yang H, Kruh-Garcia NA, Dobos KM. Purified protein derivatives of tuberculin—Past, present, and future. FEMS Immunology and Medical Microbiology. 2012;**66**(3):273. DOI: 10.1111/J.1574-695X.2012.01002.X

[104] Cho YS et al. Deciphering the proteome of the in vivo diagnostic reagent "purified protein derivative" from *Mycobacterium tuberculosis*. Proteomics. 2012;**12**(7):979-991. DOI: 10.1002/PMIC.201100544

[105] WHO operational handbook on tuberculosis. Module 3: diagnosis – rapid diagnostics for tuberculosis detection, third edition. Geneva: World Health Organization; 2024. Licence: CC BY-NC-SA 3.0 IGO

[106] Kotei E, Thirunavukarasu R. Computational techniques for the automated detection of *Mycobacterium tuberculosis* from digitized sputum smear microscopic images: A systematic review. Progress in Biophysics and Molecular Biology. 2022;**171**:4-16. DOI: 10.1016/J.PBIOMOLBIO.2022.03.004

[107] Lawn SD, Kerkhoff AD, Vogt M, Wood R. Diagnostic accuracy of a low-cost, urine antigen, point-of-care screening assay for HIV-associated pulmonary tuberculosis before antiretroviral therapy: A descriptive study. The Lancet Infectious Diseases. 2012;**12**(3):201-209. DOI: 10.1016/S1473-3099(11)70251-1

[108] Gupta-Wright A, Peters JA, Flach C, Lawn SD. Detection of lipoarabinomannan (LAM) in urine is an independent predictor of mortality risk in patients receiving treatment for HIV-associated tuberculosis in sub-Saharan Africa: A systematic review and meta-analysis. BMC Medicine. 2016;**14**(1). DOI: 10.1186/S12916-016-0603-9

[109] Olawoye IB et al. Whole genome sequencing of clinical samples reveals extensively drug resistant tuberculosis (XDR TB) strains from the Beijing lineage in Nigeria, West Africa. Scientific Reports. 2021;**11**(1):17387. DOI: 10.1038/S41598-021-96956-7

[110] *Mycobacterium tuberculosis* whole-genome sequencing and cluster investigation handbook—GOV.UK. Available from: https://www.gov.uk/government/publications/tb-strain-typing-and-cluster-investigation-handbook/mycobacterium-tuberculosis-whole-genome-sequencing-and-cluster-investigation-handbook#authors [Accessed: 8 December 2024]

[111] Cr. consortium. DNA sequencing predicts 1st-line tuberculosis drug

susceptibility profiles. The New England Journal of Medicine. 2018;**379**(15):1403. DOI: 10.1056/NEJMOA1800474

[112] Zade A, Shah S, Hirani N, Kondabagil K, Joshi A, Chatterjee A. Whole-genome sequencing of presumptive MDR-TB isolates from a tertiary healthcare setting in Mumbai. Journal of Global Antimicrobial Resistance. 2022;**31**:256-262. DOI: 10.1016/J.JGAR.2022.10.004

[113] WHO. Catalogue of mutations in *Mycobacterium tuberculosis* complex and their association with drug resistance; 2021

[114] OMS. WHO consolidated guidelines on tuberculosis. Module 3: Diagnosis-rapid diagnostics for tuberculosis detection, 2021 update. World Health Organization. 2021. Available from: https://www.who.int/publications/i/item/9789240029415;**Module 3**:1-164 [Accessed: 22 September 2024]

[115] Naidoo K, Perumal R, Ngema SL, Shunmugam L, Somboro AM. Rapid diagnosis of drug-resistant tuberculosis–opportunities and challenges. Pathogens. 2024;**13**(1). DOI: 10.3390/PATHOGENS13010027

[116] WHO. Use of targeted next-generation sequencing to detect drug-resistant tuberculosis. Available from: https://www.who.int/publications/i/item/9789240076372 [Accessed: 22 September 2024]

[117] Nusrath Unissa A, Hanna LE. Molecular mechanisms of action, resistance, detection to the first-line anti tuberculosis drugs: Rifampicin and pyrazinamide in the post whole genome sequencing era. Tuberculosis (Edinburgh, Scotland). 2017;**105**:96-107. DOI: 10.1016/J.TUBE.2017.04.008

[118] Taniguchi H et al. Rifampicin resistance and mutation of the rpoB gene in *Mycobacterium tuberculosis*. FEMS Microbiology Letters. 1996;**144**(1):103-108. DOI: 10.1111/J.1574-6968.1996.TB08515.X

[119] Brammachary U, Ramachandra V, Palavesam S, Kapalamurthy RC, Muralidhar A, Muthaiah M. Mechanisms and action of drug resistance on mycobacterium tuberculosis. Antibiotic Resistance - New Insights [Working Title]. IntechOpen; 21 Dec 2022. DOI: 10.5772/intechopen.108943

[120] Telenti A et al. The emb operon, a gene cluster of *Mycobacterium tuberculosis* involved in resistance to ethambutol. Nature Medicine. 1997;**3**(5):567-570. DOI: 10.1038/NM0597-567

[121] Cheng S, Cui Z, Li Y, Hu Z. Diagnostic accuracy of a molecular drug susceptibility testing method for the antituberculosis drug ethambutol: A systematic review and meta-analysis. Journal of Clinical Microbiology. 2014;**52**(8):2913-2924. DOI: 10.1128/JCM.00560-14

[122] Yadon AN et al. A comprehensive characterization of PncA polymorphisms that confer resistance to pyrazinamide. Nature Communications. 2017;**8**(1). DOI: 10.1038/S41467-017-00721-2

[123] Dohál M et al. Resistance patterns and transmission of mono- and polyresistant TB: Clinical impact of WGS. JAC-Antimicrobial Resistance. 2023;**5**(5). DOI: 10.1093/JACAMR/DLAD108

[124] Sterling TR. Fluoroquinolones for the treatment and prevention of multidrug-resistant tuberculosis. International Journal of Tuberculosis and Lung Disease. 2016;**20**(12):S42-S47. DOI: 10.5588/IJTLD.16.0117

[125] Chaoui I, Oudghiri A, El Mzibri M. Characterization of gyrA and gyrB mutations associated with fluoroquinolone resistance in *Mycobacterium tuberculosis* isolates from Morocco. Journal of Global Antimicrobial Resistance. 2018;**12**:171-174. DOI: 10.1016/J.JGAR.2017.10.003

[126] Kadura S et al. Systematic review of mutations associated with resistance to the new and repurposed *Mycobacterium tuberculosis* drugs bedaquiline, clofazimine, linezolid, delamanid and pretomanid. The Journal of Antimicrobial Chemotherapy. 2020;**75**(8):2031-2043. DOI: 10.1093/JAC/DKAA136

[127] Karmakar M, Rodrigues CHM, Holt KE, Dunstan SJ, Denholm J, Ascher DB. Empirical ways to identify novel Bedaquiline resistance mutations in AtpE. PLoS One. 2019;**14**(5). DOI: 10.1371/JOURNAL.PONE.0217169

[128] Degiacomi G, Sammartino JC, Sinigiani V, Marra P, Urbani A, Pasca MR. In vitro study of bedaquiline resistance in *Mycobacterium tuberculosis* multi-drug resistant clinical isolates. Frontiers in Microbiology. 2020;**11**. DOI: 10.3389/FMICB.2020.559469

[129] Pi R, Liu Q, Jiang Q, Gao Q. Characterization of linezolid-resistance-associated mutations in *Mycobacterium tuberculosis* through WGS. The Journal of Antimicrobial Chemotherapy. 2019;**74**(7):1795-1798. DOI: 10.1093/JAC/DKZ150

[130] Fujiwara M, Kawasaki M, Hariguchi N, Liu Y, Matsumoto M. Mechanisms of resistance to delamanid, a drug for *Mycobacterium tuberculosis*. Tuberculosis (Edinburgh, Scotland). 2018;**108**:186-194. DOI: 10.1016/J.TUBE.2017.12.006

[131] Manjunatha UH et al. Identification of a nitroimidazo-oxazine-specific protein involved in PA-824 resistance in *Mycobacterium tuberculosis*. Proceedings of the National Academy of Sciences of the United States of America. 2006;**103**(2):431-436. DOI: 10.1073/PNAS.0508392103

[132] Lee BM et al. Predicting nitroimidazole antibiotic resistance mutations in *Mycobacterium tuberculosis* with protein engineering. PLoS Pathogens. 2020;**16**(2). DOI: 10.1371/JOURNAL.PPAT.1008287

[133] Desjardins CA et al. Genomic and functional analyses of *Mycobacterium tuberculosis* strains implicate ald in D-cycloserine resistance. Nature Genetics. 2016;**48**(5):544-551. DOI: 10.1038/NG.3548

[134] Nakatani Y et al. Role of alanine racemase mutations in *Mycobacterium tuberculosis* d-cycloserine resistance. Antimicrobial Agents and Chemotherapy. 2017;**61**(12). DOI: 10.1128/AAC.01575-17

[135] Georghiou SB, Magana M, Garfein RS, Catanzaro DG, Catanzaro A, Rodwell TC. Evaluation of genetic mutations associated with *Mycobacterium tuberculosis* resistance to amikacin, kanamycin and capreomycin: A systematic review. PLoS One. 2012;7(3). DOI: 10.1371/JOURNAL.PONE.0033275

[136] Pandey B, Grover S, Kaur J, Grover A. Analysis of mutations leading to para-aminosalicylic acid resistance in *Mycobacterium tuberculosis*. Scientific Reports. 2019;**9**(1). DOI: 10.1038/S41598-019-48940-5

[137] Mathys V et al. Molecular genetics of para-aminosalicylic acid resistance in clinical isolates and spontaneous mutants of *Mycobacterium*

tuberculosis. Antimicrobial Agents and Chemotherapy. 2009;**53**(5):2100-2109. DOI: 10.1128/AAC.01197-08

[138] Ushtanit A, Kulagina E, Mikhailova Y, Makarova M, Safonova S, Zimenkov D. Molecular determinants of ethionamide resistance in clinical isolates of *Mycobacterium tuberculosis*. Antibiotics (Basel). 2022;**11**(2). DOI: 10.3390/ANTIBIOTICS11020133

[139] Dover LG et al. Crystal structure of the TetR/CamR family repressor *Mycobacterium tuberculosis* EthR implicated in ethionamide resistance. Journal of Molecular Biology. 2004;**340**(5):1095-1105. DOI: 10.1016/j.jmb.2004.06.003

[140] Brosch R et al. Genome plasticity of BCG and impact on vaccine efficacy. Proceedings of the National Academy of Sciences of the United States of America. 2007;**104**(13):5596-5601. DOI: 10.1073/PNAS.0700869104

[141] Tran V, Ahn SK, Ng M, Li M, Liu J. Loss of lipid virulence factors reduces the efficacy of the BCG vaccine. Scientific Reports. 2016;**6**. DOI: 10.1038/SREP29076

[142] Von Reyn CF et al. Prevention of tuberculosis in Bacille Calmette-Guérin-primed, HIV-infected adults boosted with an inactivated whole-cell mycobacterial vaccine. AIDS. 2010;**24**(5):675-685. DOI: 10.1097/QAD.0B013E3283350F1B

[143] Munseri P et al. DAR-901 vaccine for the prevention of infection with *Mycobacterium tuberculosis* among BCG-immunized adolescents in Tanzania: A randomized controlled, double-blind phase 2b trial. Vaccine. 2020;**38**(46):7239-7245. DOI: 10.1016/J.VACCINE.2020.09.055

[144] Sharma SK et al. Efficacy and safety of Mycobacterium indicus pranii as an adjunct therapy in category II pulmonary tuberculosis in a randomized trial. Scientific Reports. 2017;**7**(1). DOI: 10.1038/S41598-017-03514-1

[145] Nell AS et al. Safety, tolerability, and immunogenicity of the novel antituberculous vaccine RUTI: Randomized, placebo-controlled phase II clinical trial in patients with latent tuberculosis infection. PLoS One. 2014;**9**(2):e89612. DOI: 10.1371/JOURNAL.PONE.0089612

[146] Cardona PJ. RUTI: A new chance to shorten the treatment of latent tuberculosis infection. Tuberculosis (Edinburgh, Scotland). 2006;**86**(3-4):273-289. DOI: 10.1016/J.TUBE.2006.01.024

[147] Tang ST et al. Genome-based in silico identification of new *Mycobacterium tuberculosis* antigens activating polyfunctional CD8+ T cells in human tuberculosis. Journal of Immunology. 2011;**186**(2):1068-1080. DOI: 10.4049/JIMMUNOL.1002212

[148] Lewinsohn DM et al. Human *Mycobacterium tuberculosis* CD8 T cell antigens/epitopes identified by a proteomic peptide library. PLoS One. 2013;**8**(6). DOI: 10.1371/JOURNAL.PONE.0067016

[149] WHO. TB-trials. Available from: https://tbtrialtrack.who.int/#/ [Accessed: 30 September 2024]

[150] StopTB Partnership. BNT164b1—Working Group on New TB Vaccines. Available from: https://newtbvaccines.org/vaccine/bnt164b1/ [Accessed: 30 September 2024]

[151] WHO. Preferred product characteristics for therapeutic vaccines

to improve tuberculosis treatment outcomes. Available from: https://iris.who.int/handle/10665/330448 [Accessed: 30 September 2024]

[152] Lai R, Ogunsola AF, Rakib T, Behar SM. Key advances in vaccine development for tuberculosis—Success and challenges. npj Vaccines. 2023;**8**(1). DOI: 10.1038/S41541-023-00750-7

[153] Yang Y, Chen YZ, Xia T. Optimizing antigen selection for the development of tuberculosis vaccines. Cell Insight. 2024;**3**(3):100163. DOI: 10.1016/J.CELLIN.2024.100163

[154] Dijkman K et al. A protective, single-visit TB vaccination regimen by co-administration of a subunit vaccine with BCG. npj Vaccines. 2023;**8**(1). DOI: 10.1038/S41541-023-00666-2

[155] ClinicalTrials.gov Registry. Study Details | First-in-Human Trial of the Novel Tuberculosis Vaccine Candidate, H107e/CAF®10b | ClinicalTrials.gov. Available from: https://clinicaltrials.gov/study/NCT06050356?intr=H107&rank=1 [Accessed: 2 October 2024]

[156] Bhargava A et al. Nutritional supplementation to prevent tuberculosis incidence in household contacts of patients with pulmonary tuberculosis in India (RATIONS): A field-based, open-label, cluster-randomised, controlled trial. Lancet. 2023;**402**(10402):627-640. DOI: 10.1016/S0140-6736(23)01231-X

[157] Sinha P et al. Food for thought: Addressing undernutrition to end tuberculosis. The Lancet Infectious Diseases. 2021;**21**(10):e318-e325. DOI: 10.1016/S1473-3099(20)30792-1

Section 3

Diagnosis and Treatment

Chapter 6

Challenges in the Diagnosis of Tuberculosis and Non-Tuberculosis Mycobacteria

Radha Gopalaswamy, Gowsalya Saminathan, Vasudevan Manoharan and Siva Kumar Shanmugam

Abstract

Tuberculosis (TB) caused by *Mycobacterium tuberculosis* (MTB) is one of the oldest diseases known to humanity, with evidence of its existence dating back thousands of years. Despite the availability of effective treatments, TB causes morbidity and mortality globally, with special reference to low- and middle-income countries (LMICs). In recent years, advancements in molecular diagnostics have transformed the landscape of TB detection. Nucleic acid amplification tests (NAAT) techniques such as polymerase chain reaction (PCR) have rapidly emerged and are well developed, offering timely and accurate identification of MTB. This chapter aims to provide a comprehensive overview of the traditional and modern diagnostic methods in clinical laboratories for MTB detection, exploring the challenges faced in TB diagnosis and the implications for public health. By understanding the intricacies of TB diagnostics, we can better address the ongoing global challenge posed by this ancient yet persistent disease, ultimately working toward a TB-free world.

Keywords: *Mycobacterium tuberculosis* (MTB), global health, molecular diagnostics, nucleic acid amplification tests (NAAT), TB diagnosis challenges

1. Introduction

Mycobacterium tuberculosis (MTB), a pathogenic bacterium, is the causative organism of tuberculosis (TB), which has been a significant public health concern for centuries as an infectious disease. TB is one of the oldest diseases known to humanity, with evidence of its existence dating back thousands of years [1]. Despite the availability of effective treatments, TB causes morbidity and mortality globally, with special reference to low- and middle-income countries (LMICs) [2]. In 2022, an estimated 10.6 million people fell ill with tuberculosis, with 7.5 million newly diagnosed cases of TB globally. Despite increased diagnosis and treatment, an estimated 1.3 million deaths were caused by TB in 2022 [3].

TB bacilli can be transmitted as droplet nuclei residues of dried respiratory droplets. A droplet nucleus that contains 1–10 TB bacilli is 1–5 μm in diameter. These droplets can remain in the air for several hours and can be inhaled into the alveoli [4, 5]. When

MTB is inhaled, alveolar macrophages kill the TB bacilli. When humans are infected with MTB, 10% of infected hosts progress to active TB disease, and the remaining 90% sustain Latent TB Infection (LTBI) [4–6]. Extrapulmonary (EP) TB occurs either as primary (at the site of initial infection) or secondary (disseminated) infection due to hematogenous or lymphatic spread of bacteria from the primary organ, reactivation of LTBI, ingestion of infected sputum, or spread locally from adjacent organ. EP-TB can occur at various sites in the body: the brain, eye, mouth, tongue, spine, bones, muscles, skin, lymph nodes of the neck, pleura, pericardium, gastrointestinal, peritoneum, and the genitourinary system as a primary and/or disseminated disease [7, 8]. Apart from tuberculosis, there are 190 nontuberculous mycobacteria (NTM) species, which poses a huge challenge to diagnosis and treatment. Most NTMs are primarily acquired from the environment and, though they primarily affect the lungs, can cause extra pulmonary infections or disease [7, 9].

Historically, the diagnosis of TB relied on traditional methods such as microscopy, culture, and the tuberculin skin test (TST) [10]. While quick and cost-effective, microscopy has limitations in sensitivity and specificity, particularly in cases of extra pulmonary TB or in patients with low bacterial loads. Culture techniques, considered the gold standard for TB diagnosis, can take weeks to yield results, delaying treatment initiation [11]. Although useful for identifying previous exposure to MTB, the TST cannot differentiate between latent and active TB and may yield false-positive results in vaccinated individuals [12]. Diagnosis of NTM is challenging, though microscopy and culture are considered gold standards for NTM diagnosis. Molecular methods for NTM diagnosis offer rapid and conclusive diagnosis for at least a few common NTM species [7].

In recent years, advancements in molecular diagnostics have transformed the landscape of TB detection [13]. Techniques such as polymerase chain reaction (PCR) and nucleic acid amplification tests (NAATs) have emerged, offering rapid and accurate identification of MTB [14]. These methods enhance sensitivity and specificity and allow for the detection of drug-resistant strains, which is critical for effective treatment. The introduction of rapid diagnostic tests has the potential to significantly reduce the time to diagnosis, enabling timely treatment and reducing transmission rates [15]. Despite these advancements, challenges remain in the diagnosis and management of TB. Access to quality diagnostic services is limited in many LMIC settings with a high TB burden. Additionally, the complexities of differentiating between latent and active TB, as well as the potential for false-positive and false-negative results, complicate clinical decision-making [16]. Furthermore, handling MTB in clinical laboratories necessitates strict adherence to safety protocols to prevent accidental exposure and transmission.

This chapter aims to provide a comprehensive overview of the clinical laboratory diagnostics for *Mycobacterium tuberculosis*, exploring traditional and modern diagnostic methods, the challenges faced in TB diagnosis, and the implications for public health. By understanding the intricacies of TB diagnostics, we can better address the ongoing global challenge posed by this ancient yet persistent disease, ultimately working toward a TB-free world.

2. Laboratory diagnoses of MTB

Laboratory tuberculosis (TB) diagnosis is essential for confirming infection, determining its severity, and identifying drug resistance. TB, caused by *Mycobacterium*

Criteria	Smear Microscopy	Solid Culture/ DST	Liquid Culture/DST	GeneXpert MTB/RIF	Truenat MTB-RIF	Line Probe Assay (LPA)	tNGS	WGS
Principle	Phenotypic detection	Phenotypic detection	Phenotypic detection	Genotypic detection	Genotypic detection	Genotypic detection	Genotypic detection	Genotypic detection
Biosafety Level	Low	Medium	High	Low	Low	Medium	Medium	High
Turnaround Time	1–2 hours	2–8 weeks	7–42 days	2 hours	1–2 hours	1–2 days	2–3 days	2–3 weeks (indirect) 2–3 days (direct)
Limit of Detection	5000–10,000 AFB/ mL	10–100 CFU/ mL	10–100 CFU/ mL	131 CFU /mL	100 CFU /mL	10,000 CFU/ mL	NA	NA
Drug Resistance Detection	None	All drugs by pDST	All drugs by pDST	Only RIF resistance	Only RIF resistance	FL and SL drugs	All drugs	All drugs
Infrastructure Requirements	Minimal	Moderate	Advanced lab and equipment set up	Requires specialized equipment	Portable with minmal lab set up	Advanced molecular lab	Portable system available	Advanced molecular lab
Portability	Yes	No	No	Yes	Yes	No	Yes	No

Table 1.
Key features of diagnostic tests.

tuberculosis, can be challenging to diagnose due to its slow-growing nature and varied clinical presentation. The key features of the conventional diagnostic tests have been recorded in **Table 1**.

2.1 Staining and smear microscopy

Staining procedures are essential in diagnosing MTB and other mycobacterial species. Due to the unique characteristics of mycobacterial cell walls, which are rich in mycolic acids, conventional staining methods such as Gram staining are ineffective [17]. Instead, specialized staining techniques are employed to visualize mycobacteria under a microscope, allowing their identification in clinical specimens. Staining of mycobacteria shows bacillary loads usually indicated as smear grades of 1+, 2+, and 3+ [18]. Although staining is rapid, it fails to differentiate TB from NTM diseases/infections, and so far, no staining technique can differentiate TB from NTM unless complemented with other tests.

2.1.1 Acid-fast staining

The most widely used staining method for mycobacteria is acid-fast staining, which exploits the unique properties of the mycobacterial cell wall [19]. The two primary acid-fast staining techniques are the Ziehl-Neelsen and Kinyoun stains [20]. In the Ziehl-Neelsen stain, the slide is heat-fixed and stained with carbol fuchsin dye, while in the Kinyoun stain, carbol fuchsin contains a higher concentration of phenol, allowing for better dye penetration without heat and ensuring that the bacteria adhere to the slide. Decolorization with acid-alcohol followed by methylene blue staining shows acid-fast bacilli (AFB) as bright red rods against a blue background [21]. The Kinyoun stain is considered less sensitive than the Ziehl-Neelsen method but is easier to perform, making it suitable for laboratories with limited resources [22].

2.1.2 Fluorescent staining

Fluorescent staining techniques, such as the auramine-rhodamine stain, are also used to detect mycobacteria. Once the smear is prepared and air-dried, the slide is stained with a mixture of auramine O and rhodamine B, which binds to the mycobacterial cell wall. The slide is rinsed with acid-alcohol to remove excess dye and examined under a fluorescent microscope, where mycobacteria appear as bright yellow-green rods against a dark background. Fluorescent staining is more sensitive than traditional acid-fast staining and allows for examining a larger number of fields under lower magnification, increasing the likelihood of detecting mycobacteria [23].

2.2 Culture

Mycobacteria are classified as slow-growing organisms, with MTB requiring approximately 15 to 40 days to form visible colonies in culture [24, 25]. This slow growth is attributed to the high lipid content of their cell walls, which contain mycolic acids. Mycobacteria are also classified as aerobic organisms, necessitating the presence of oxygen for growth [26]. Understanding these characteristics is essential for developing effective culturing techniques.

2.2.1 Culture media for mycobacteria

The choice of culture medium is crucial for mycobacteria's successful isolation and growth. Several types of media are used, including solid and liquid media, each with advantages and disadvantages. Solid media, such as egg-based media (Lowenstein-Jensen medium) and agar-based media (Middlebrook 7H10 and 7H11), are commonly used for culturing mycobacteria [27]. Lowenstein-Jensen Medium is an egg-based medium rich in nutrients and provides a solid surface for colony formation. It is particularly useful for isolating MTB from clinical specimens. However, this medium's growth rate is slower than broth media, often taking 18–24 days for visible colonies to appear [28]. Middlebrook 7H10 and 7H11 Media are agar-based media designed specifically for mycobacterial growth and contain various nutrients, including glycerol and oleic acid. They support faster growth of MTB compared to egg-based media, with colonies typically appearing within 10–12 days [29]. Liquid media, such as Middlebrook 7H9 broth and BACTEC MGIT (Mycobacterial Growth Indicator Tube), are increasingly used for culturing mycobacteria due to their rapidly recovering organisms. Middlebrook 7H9 broth supports the growth of mycobacteria in a liquid format, allowing for continuous growth monitoring. It is often supplemented with oleic acid, albumin, and dextrose to enhance growth. The BACTEC MGIT System is a semi-automated broth culture system using fluorometric methods to detect mycobacterial growth. The system continuously monitors the culture for changes in fluorescence, allowing for rapid detection of MTB, often within 7–14 days. The MGIT system has a sensitivity of 88–93% for detecting mycobacterial growth [30].

2.2.2 Culturing techniques

Clinical specimens, such as sputum, bronchoalveolar lavage fluid, or tissue biopsies, are collected from patients suspected of having TB or other mycobacterial infections [31]. Proper collection techniques are essential to minimize contamination. Specimens may undergo a decontamination process to eliminate non-mycobacterial contaminants. Common decontamination agents include sodium hydroxide or N-acetylcysteine, which help reduce contaminants' bacterial load while preserving mycobacterial viability [16]. To prevent contamination, the decontaminated specimen is inoculated onto the chosen culture medium (solid or liquid) using sterile techniques. For solid media, the specimen is streaked onto the surface, while for liquid media, it is added directly to the broth. Cultures are incubated at 35–37°C in an atmosphere containing 5–10% CO_2. The incubation period may vary depending on the media used, with solid media requiring longer periods for colony formation. Cultures are monitored regularly for signs of growth. In solid media, colonies are examined for characteristic morphology, while in liquid media, changes in fluorescence or turbidity indicate growth.

2.2.3 MGIT drug susceptibility testing (DST)

It involves cultivating *Mycobacterium tuberculosis* in a liquid culture within MGIT tubes equipped with a fluorescent oxygen sensor. The process uses two types of tubes: one containing no drugs (control) and another with specific anti-TB drugs. As bacteria grow, they consume oxygen, which alters the fluorescence detected by the system. If the bacteria are susceptible to the drug, their growth is inhibited, resulting in lower fluorescence in the drug-containing tube compared to the control. If the bacteria are resistant, growth continues despite the drug, leading to similar fluorescence levels in both tubes. The automated MGIT system monitors these fluorescence changes to assess drug susceptibility based on the growth patterns. The drug susceptibility testing is based on the principle of proportionate sensitivity test [32].

The 1% proportionate sensitivity test assesses *Mycobacterium tuberculosis* resistance to anti-TB drugs by comparing bacterial growth on media with and without the drug. In this test, a bacterial isolate is cultured on solid media, with one set containing the drug at a 1% concentration and the other set serving as a control without the drug. After incubation, the growth of colonies on both media is compared. If the proportion of colonies growing on the drug-containing medium is 1% or more of the control, the strain is classified as resistant; if it is less than 1%, the strain is considered susceptible. This test helps determine the effectiveness of the drug against the TB strain. The critical concentrations of the drugs used in the TB regimen, according to the Technical Report on critical concentrations for drug susceptibility testing, have been tabulated in **Table 2** [33].

Although the same culturing technique can be used for NTM, it is well known that using p-nitro benzoic acid in solid or liquid media can discriminate NTM from MTB. Inclusion of PNB retards the growth of MTB but promotes NTM growth differentially, identifying culture positive for NTM. The time to detection for NTM in PNB containing liquid media is 7 days, and solid media is 28 days [34, 35].

2.3 Nucleic acid amplification tests

Nucleic Acid Amplification Tests (NAATs) have transformed the landscape of tuberculosis (TB) diagnostics by providing a fast, accurate, and highly sensitive method for detecting *Mycobacterium tuberculosis*, the causative agent of TB [36]. These tests utilize sophisticated molecular techniques to amplify and identify specific

Type	Drugs	Critical Concentration	Solvent
First-Line drugs	Isoniazid (INH)	0.1 µg/mL	Dimethyl sulfoxide (DMSO)
	Rifampicin (RIF)	1.0 µg/mL	Dimethyl sulfoxide (DMSO)
	Ethambutol (EMB)	2.0 µg/mL	Dimethyl sulfoxide (DMSO)
	Pyrazinamide (PZA)	10.0 µg/mL	Dimethyl sulfoxide (DMSO)
Second-Line drugs	Amikacin	1.0 µg/mL	Water
	Capreomycin	2.5 µg/mL	Water
	Kanamycin	2.5 µg/mL	Water
	Streptomycin	1.0 µg/mL	Water
	Ethionamide	5.0 µg/mL	Dimethyl sulfoxide (DMSO)
	Prothionamide	2.5 µg/mL	Dimethyl sulfoxide (DMSO)
	Linezolid	1.0 µg/mL	Dimethyl sulfoxide (DMSO)
	Clofazimine	1.0 µg/mL	Dimethyl sulfoxide (DMSO)
Newer Drugs	Bedaquiline	1.0 µg/mL	Dimethyl sulfoxide (DMSO)
	Delamanid	0.06 First-Line µg/mL	Dimethyl sulfoxide (DMSO)

Table 2.
Critical concentration and solvent used for each drug in TB treatment.

genetic markers unique to the TB bacterium, which allows for quicker and more precise diagnoses compared to conventional methods such as sputum smear microscopy and culture, which are often slower and less accurate [37]. While low complexity NAATs like the GeneXpert MTB/RIF and Truenat MTB-RIF identify TB and rifampicin resistance within 2 hours, a moderate-complexity NAAT-like line probe assay offers detection of resistance to first- and second-line drugs.

2.3.1 GeneXpert MTB/RIF

GeneXpert MTB/RIF is a cartridge-based system that utilizes the NAAT technique to detect the presence of MTB DNA and mutations in the rifampicin resistance-associated *rpoB* gene within a 2-hour turnaround time [38]. The GeneXpert procedure for TB diagnosis involves collecting a clinical sample, sputum, or extra pulmonary specimen suitably prepared for the test and mixing it with a sample reagent to liquefy and decontaminate the sample. This mixture is then transferred into a GeneXpert cartridge, which contains all the necessary reagents for PCR. The cartridge is placed into the GeneXpert machine, where the system automatically processes the sample, amplifies the MTB DNA, and simultaneously detects mutations indicating rifampicin resistance. The results, indicating TB presence and drug resistance, are displayed on the machine within 2 hours, allowing for quick and accurate diagnosis. Although GeneXpert performs well in detecting rifampicin resistance with high sensitivity and specificity during initial multicentre evaluations, some studies have reported false-positive rifampicin resistance in regions with low prevalence of resistance, as detected through *rpoB* gene sequencing and other methods [39, 40]. The bacillary load is indicated as Very low, Low, Medium, and High when there is a positive test for MTB. GeneXpert can be used with sputum and various extra pulmonary samples, including stool, pus, tissue, nodes, and fluids, as recommended by WHO.

2.3.2 Truenat MTB-RIF

Truenat is a molecular diagnostic platform based on polymerase chain reaction (PCR) technology. It detects the presence of MTB DNA in clinical samples by amplifying specific target sequences of the bacterial genome. Additionally, Truenat can identify resistance to rifampicin, one of the first-line drugs for TB treatment, making it useful for diagnosing drug-resistant TB (DR-TB) [41]. The system is designed for rapid, point-of-care testing, particularly in resource-limited settings. Amplification and detection of MTB are done using real-time micro-PCR technology. Within 1–2 hours, the device provides results on its screen, indicating the presence of MTB along with the bacillary load in terms of CFU/mL. Following the detection of MTB, rifampicin testing is carried out and uses an in-built melt curve analysis for rifampicin detection [42]. Truenat MTB testing can be performed with sputum and other non-sputum extrapulmonary samples [43].

2.3.3 Line probe assay (LPA)

A line probe assay is a DNA strip-based test employed to determine the drug resistance profile of an MTBC strain. This profiling is done by analyzing the pattern of DNA amplicons that bind to immobilized oligonucleotides on a test strip that acts as a probe [44]. These probes target the most common resistance-associated mutations. LPAs are WHO-approved tests for rapid detection of drug resistance to first- and second-line drugs. The assay identifies mutations by emitting a colorimetric signal, indicating resistance to isoniazid or rifampicin in the case of First-line LPA and fluoroquinolones and second-line injectable in the case of Second-Line LPA [45]. The line probe assay (LPA) allows for the detection of specific genetic sequences associated with MTB and drug resistance mutations. The results are visualized as lines on the membrane, indicating the presence of MTB and the drug resistance pattern, typically within 1–2 days. LPAs effectively detect drug-resistant MTB strains in smear-positive samples and offer high diagnostic accuracy even in smear-negative TB cases [46, 47].

2.3.4 Real-time PCR

Real-time PCR-based kits are available for differentiating MTB from NTM using different sample types, including sputum and non-sputum-based EP samples. Genedia MTB/NTM and Anyplex plus MTB/NTM have a sensitivity of 73.9% each and specificity of 100% and 99.3%, respectively, offering a rapid diagnosis of NTM [48, 49].

2.3.5 Next-generation sequencing

The use of Next-Generation Sequencing (NGS) to assess comprehensive drug resistance-associated mutations is a promising tool for clinical care. Next-Generation Sequencing (NGS) is a high-throughput method for simultaneous sequencing of multiple genes to compare with reference sequence libraries [50, 51]. NGS applications encompass targeted NGS (NGS) and WGS, with the former focusing on specific targets of genomic regions, while in WGS, the entire genome is sequenced, including the drug resistance genes. Both techniques have similar steps, starting from the (a) preparation of DNA from bacterial cultures or clinical specimens, (b) library preparation involving multiplexing of samples, (c) use of a sequencing platform where multiple DNA fragments are sequenced in parallel, and (d) bioinformatics approach to map the individual reads to the reference genome. WGS requires culture as the preferred starting material, while tNGS can be standardized for use with direct clinical specimens [50, 51]. WGS and tNGS have different platforms with either elaborate, sophisticated Illumina platforms or the portable Minion system. This system could use in-house or commercial primers to include the identification of NTM [52–54].

3. Challenges in tuberculosis diagnosis

3.1 Technical challenges

Diagnosing tuberculosis presents several technical challenges due to the disease's complex nature and the limitations of current diagnostic methods. The barriers have been elaborated as follows.

3.1.1 Sample type

Common specimens include sputum, bronchoalveolar lavage fluid, and tissue biopsies, which can have different diagnostic values from smear and staining. The quality of the sample is paramount; inadequate or poorly collected specimens can lead to false-negative results [55]. Besides, preparation of the smear and the choice of staining technique can also pose challenges. Interpreting stained smears requires expertise and experience. The presence of AFB must be distinguished from artifacts, debris, and other non-specific staining. Misinterpretation can lead to incorrect conclusions about the presence or absence of mycobacteria. Additionally, the subjective nature of microscopy means that results can vary between different observers, leading to inconsistencies in diagnosis. In EP-TB samples, it is impossible to get multiple samples, and hence, smear and staining as a conclusive test is not recommended. Smear and staining are performed only after there is availability of a sample for better confirmatory tests.

Among NAAT, the quality and consistency of sputum samples can vary, affecting the efficiency of the test, especially if the samples are too viscous or contain inhibitors [56]. Proper handling and storage of reagents are critical to maintain their effectiveness, and any deviations in processing time can impact the accuracy of the results. Skilled operators are essential for accurate sample preparation; inadequate training can lead to errors. Additionally, handling infectious sputum samples requires stringent biosafety measures to protect laboratory staff and prevent cross-contamination. Addressing these challenges is crucial for ensuring the reliability and accuracy of the GeneXpert diagnostic system. Sample types like EP-TB or pediatric samples, though offered upfront NAAT, depending on the sample type and quality, the diagnostic value of NAAT is a challenge. Wherever the sample type is proper and adequate, it is a good point-of-care (POC) test for TB diagnosis.

Sample preparation for the line probe assay (LPA) involves several challenges, including ensuring that the sputum samples are properly processed to extract and purify DNA effectively [55]. Variations in sample quality or incomplete processing can lead to inaccurate results. The amplification and hybridization steps require precise handling of reagents and adherence to protocols to avoid contamination and ensure accurate detection of *Mycobacterium tuberculosis* and drug resistance mutations. While NGS offers a one-stop solution for comprehensive drug resistance profiling, culture is the preferred sample choice for WGS in higher labs. tNGS can be performed from clinical specimens but requires training in handling and processing samples and interpretation of results.

3.1.2 Bacillary load

Pediatric TB and extra pulmonary TB pose a challenge, with the former well-known being unable to expectorate good quality sputum. Secondly, in extra pulmonary TB or patients with compromised immune systems (PL-HIV), the number of mycobacteria may be insufficient for detection [57]. AFB may be present in very low quantities, making it difficult to visualize them in a smear. This low sensitivity can result in false-negative results, delaying diagnosis and treatment. Low bacillary load poses a significant challenge for NAAT, as the test relies on detecting DNA from *Mycobacterium tuberculosis* (MTB) at least from 100 to 131 CFU/mL between GeneXpert and Truenat [58]. In cases of low bacterial count, such as in early TB infection, pediatric TB, or immunocompromised patients, NAAT's sensitivity may be reduced, leading to false-negative results. The limited number of bacteria present can result in insufficient amplification of MTB DNA during the PCR process, making it harder for the system to accurately detect the disease. Besides MTB testing, low bacillary load samples offer inconclusive results with rifampicin resistance, thus making upfront UDST impossible.

Although LPA is highly sensitive in detecting TB and drug-resistant mutations, it is restricted only to smear-positive samples [46]. With a minimum bacterial load required to produce sufficient DNA for amplification and hybridization, and in samples with very few bacilli, such as those from patients with paucibacillary TB, the assay might depend on indirect LPA through cultures to detect the pathogen or drug resistance. When the culture becomes negative or contaminated, there are no further results available for first-line or second-line drugs beyond NAAT. Besides, the number of laboratories performing LPA is minimal and is much less than a point-of-care testing (POCT) like NAAT. Although WGS requires a higher quality and quantity of sample, it yields a comprehensive drug resistance profile. However, with tNGS, low quality and quantity of sample DNA from direct sputum can be used since an amplification step is involved. However, currently, it is restricted a to fairly high bacillary load as identified by either smear grades or CT or CFUs/mL indicated by real-time PCR for confirmation of MTB in the sample.

3.1.2.1 NTM identification

The presence of nontuberculous mycobacteria (NTM) in clinical specimens can complicate the interpretation of smear results. NTMs can also appear as AFB, leading to potential misidentification. Differentiating between MTB and NTMs based solely on smear results is challenging, as both groups can exhibit similar staining characteristics. This issue underscores the need for further identification methods, such as culture or molecular techniques, to confirm the presence of specific mycobacterial species.

NAAT, like GeneXpert MTB/RIF or Truenat MTB-RIF, is designed specifically to detect MTB and rifampicin resistance, but NTM can still pose challenges [59–61]. While GeneXpert generally does not detect NTM, mixed infections or contamination with NTM can complicate the sample interpretation and potentially cause false-negative or ambiguous results. Recently, however, real-time PCR-based kits like Genedia MTB/NTM and Anyplex plus MTB/NTM are available to identify NTM [48]. Identifying an NTM-causing disease over its role as a commensal/colonizer requires clinical correlation and the right interpretation of test results. It is highly recommended to repeat the test with a duplicate sample wherever possible. Hains LPA Genotype Mycobacterium CM and AS assays are designed to identify common and associated species of NTM and DR LPA for identifying drug resistance in some NTM species of Mycobacterium avium complex (MAC) and detect resistance to macrolides and aminoglycosides in nontuberculous mycobacteria (NTM). Besides that, tNGS kits commercially available can detect NTM from nearly 120 species using different pipelines commercially provided for the bioinformatics analysis. Similarly, NTM can be detected when WGS is done from a culture, enabling further profiling if a suitable pipeline is created.

3.1.3 Contamination

Contamination is a significant concern in the culture of mycobacteria. Non-mycobacterial organisms can outgrow mycobacteria in culture, complicating isolation and leading to false-positive results. Contaminants can arise from various sources, including the environment, laboratory equipment, and specimens. Implementing effective decontamination procedures is essential, but these methods must be carefully optimized to avoid harming the viability of mycobacteria. The contamination challenge underscores the importance of maintaining high laboratory practice standards and implementing robust quality control measures. The viability of mycobacteria in clinical specimens can be affected by various factors, including the method of specimen collection, transport conditions, and storage [62, 63]. Mycobacteria are sensitive to environmental conditions, and improper handling can lead to a decrease in viability. For instance, exposure to extreme temperatures or prolonged transport times can compromise the specimen's integrity, making it more challenging to culture viable organisms. Ensuring proper specimen handling and transport is crucial for successful culture outcomes.

3.1.4 Biosafety and waste disposal

With smear and staining, although phenol is required for disposing of the sputum containers, there are no specific requirements for PPE other than gowns or lab coats. With NAAT and LPA, lab coats, masks, and gloves are required to process the sample. Apart from phenol, sodium hypochlorite is required to discard the chips in Truenat and the LPA facility to dispose of tubes and strips. To prevent cross-contamination, sodium hypochlorite is mandatory for cleaning work surfaces in NAAT and LPA facilities. Regarding MGIT, back closure gowns with N95 masks, gloves, shoe covers, and hair covers are required. Proper biowaste management with autoclaves is required to dispose of the waste from BSC and BSL3 facilities. WGS requirements are similar to culture, and for tNGS, it is similar to DNA extraction as seen in LPA. No additional requirements or waste disposal is required.

3.2 Operational challenges

Operational challenges in tuberculosis (TB) diagnosis pose significant barriers to effective disease control, particularly in high-burden regions. These challenges include inadequate laboratory infrastructure, limited access to diagnostic tools like GeneXpert, and shortages of trained personnel. Additionally, logistical issues such as delayed sample transportation, poor quality control in testing procedures, and insufficient integration of diagnostic services within health systems further complicate the diagnostic process [64]. Furthermore, socioeconomic factors, such as patients' distance from healthcare facilities and the stigma surrounding the disease, can lead to delayed diagnosis and treatment. Addressing these operational challenges is critical to improving TB diagnosis and ultimately reducing the global TB burden. Some of the major operational challenges are.

3.2.1 Sample transportation

The primary challenge in sample transport is preserving the viability of mycobacteria as well as preventing the growth of other flora. Depending on the resource setting, it requires an intensive focus on sample transportation—testing capacity of the referral lab, maintenance of patient confidentiality during transit, means of sample transport, and scheduling of transport frequency. The means of transport depend on the terrain, distance, and resources of the sample collection area [65]. Challenges in sample transportation include delay in transportation, lack of adequate packaging material, improper packaging and lack of maintenance of proper temperature, leakage, missing samples, and mismatch referral forms, all leading to improper transportation to the lab, leading to failure of the sample diagnosis [66, 67].

3.2.2 High cost

Although smear microscopy offers the least budget for starting smear and staining of mycobacteria with sustenance, it provides minimal information on the presence of mycobacteria, necessitating a higher-level test to be required for confirmation [68]. The high cost associated with the NAAT system presents a significant challenge to its widespread implementation in tuberculosis (TB) diagnostics. The initial investment required to purchase the GeneXpert or a Truenat machine is substantial, which can be a major barrier for many healthcare facilities, especially in LMICs. In addition to the initial cost, the recurring expense of purchasing specialized single-use cartridges/chips for each test further compounds the financial burden. These chips or cartridges are expensive and create ongoing operational costs that strain already limited healthcare budgets [69]. In many regions, the cost of the NAAT system is often mitigated by external funding sources such as international aid [70]. LPAs face challenges due to their high cost and technical complexity. Establishing an LPA testing facility requires a substantial financial investment in specialized equipment, including thermocyclers, hybridization ovens, and automated systems for detecting genetic mutations. The cost of reagents used in LPAs is also significant, and ongoing consumable expenses can strain budgets, especially in low-resource settings [71]. MGIT960 instrument cost and requirement of a BSL3 facility for liquid culture handling can be expensive and require sophistication. Concerning NGS, either WGS or tNGS requires a huge financial investment initially and sufficient samples to be included in one batch [72]. Procuring sequencing instruments and reagents with short expiry requires planning and optimal utilization at the facility.

3.2.3 Infrastructure

While staining and microscopy do not demand bigger infrastructure requirements, the GeneXpert system must pose significant challenges, especially in settings where resources are scarce and essential infrastructure may be insufficient or absent. While the GeneXpert machine is relatively easy to operate, it still requires a consistent and uninterrupted power supply to function properly. In many LMICs, particularly in rural or isolated areas, the electricity supply can be unstable, with frequent power outages and fluctuations. These disruptions can interrupt testing processes, damage sensitive equipment, or result in incomplete or inaccurate results, ultimately impacting the quality of patient care. Furthermore, the GeneXpert system requires a controlled environment, especially concerning temperature and humidity, to perform optimally [73]. The machine and its cartridges are vulnerable to extreme temperatures, commonly encountered in tropical or desert regions where the climate can exceed the recommended operational range for the equipment. Without proper climate control measures, such as air conditioning or temperature-regulated storage, the machine's accuracy and performance can suffer, leading to diagnostic errors. Although Truenat is designed for decentralized settings, Truenat chips and reagents are sensitive to temperature variations [36]. Maintaining the required temperature for reagents is challenging in regions with extreme climates, such as tropical or desert areas. Reagents may degrade without proper cold chain logistics, leading to inaccurate or unreliable results. Meeting the refrigeration needs can be difficult in areas lacking adequate infrastructure. The successful implementation of LPAs depends on having the necessary laboratory infrastructure, which is a significant challenge in many settings. LPAs require a Biosafety Level 2 laboratory with designated areas for

DNA extraction, amplification, and post-amplification processes to prevent cross-contamination [74]. Many healthcare facilities lack such advanced infrastructure, especially in low- and middle-income countries. Maintaining consistent power supply and environmental controls, such as temperature and humidity regulation, is also crucial for the accurate functioning of LPA equipment. In regions with unstable power grids or extreme environmental conditions, upholding these standards can be challenging, potentially disrupting testing and compromising result reliability. The substantial investment required for these infrastructure needs often exceeds the financial capacity of many healthcare systems in resource-limited settings, limiting the widespread adoption of LPAs. With the MGIT 960 instrument, there is an elaborate requirement for BSC, uninterrupted power supply, and air conditioning. Besides, reagents and supplements need to be stored in the refrigerator or cold room, and a printer is needed to enable the use of the machine readouts for diagnosis. For WGS or tNGS, based on the platform used, it may require sophistication. The Illumina platform requires temperature and humidity to be maintained as per manufacturer instructions. Besides, there is a need for computers with huge space for data storage and processing to run bioinformatic pipelines for WGS or tNGS.

3.2.4 Supply chain management

Effective supply chain management is vital for deploying and operating the GeneXpert cartridges, Truenat chips, LPA kits, and MGIT 960 consumable systems in tuberculosis (TB) diagnostics. It ensures that materials such as cartridges, reagents, and other consumables are consistently available in the right quantities to meet testing needs. Cartridges must be imported and distributed to various testing locations, and any disruption in the supply chain, such as shipping delays, customs clearance issues, or logistical difficulties within the country, leads to stockouts. Stockouts hinder the ability of healthcare facilities to conduct tests, delaying TB diagnoses and treatment, which can have serious public health repercussions [75]. Transportation logistics also represent a significant challenge. In many LMICs, transportation infrastructure is often inadequate, with poorly maintained roads, limited access to remote regions, and unreliable transport services. These factors can slow the delivery of cartridges and other essential supplies to healthcare facilities, particularly in rural or hard-to-reach areas.

Additionally, maintaining the integrity of these supplies during transit is crucial, as cartridges and reagents are sensitive to environmental conditions such as temperature and humidity. Poor transportation conditions may compromise the quality of these materials, leading to inaccurate test results or the need to discard compromised supplies, further straining limited resources. LPA for NTM is not done routinely, and the calculation of adequate supply with usage within the expiration period should be appropriately planned. Storage is another critical aspect of supply chain management, and ensuring proper storage conditions, especially temperature control, is essential to maintaining the effectiveness of the cartridges. In many regions, however, there is a lack of storage facilities with climate control capabilities. This shortfall necessitates further investment in infrastructure, such as cold chain systems or temperature-controlled storage units, to ensure supplies are preserved in optimal conditions until use.

Accurate forecasting and inventory management are also key components of GeneXpert's supply chain management. Predicting the demand for cartridges and other supplies can be difficult, particularly when TB prevalence and healthcare facility capacity fluctuate. Without precise forecasting, facilities may overstock—leading to wastage due to expiration—or understock, causing shortages and interruptions in testing services. Implementing effective inventory management systems is essential to track stock levels, monitor usage patterns, and ensure timely reordering of supplies. For the WGS and tNGS systems with access at only higher labs, supply chain management relies on the lab team for the activities and contingency plan for any short supplies. Failure of the storage space to maintain temperature or instrument delays should be well planned out.

3.2.5 Limited detection scope

Smear microscopy has a poor scope of differentiating mycobacterial species and does not provide information on drug resistance [76]. However, the NAAT system represents a significant advancement in TB diagnostics; it has limitations regarding its detection scope, which can impact comprehensive TB management. The GeneXpert MTB/RIF or the Truenat MTB-RIF assay, the most frequently used NAAT POCT test, is designed to detect *Mycobacterium tuberculosis* and resistance to rifampicin, a primary anti-TB medication. Although detecting rifampicin resistance is vital for identifying multidrug-resistant TB (MDR-TB), the test's focus on this single drug means it does not detect resistance to other first-line or second-line TB drugs, such as Isoniazid, Ethambutol, Fluoroquinolones. This limitation necessitates additional testing with other methods, such as line probe assays or culture-based drug susceptibility tests, to fully determine the resistance profile of the TB strain, which can delay the initiation of appropriate treatment. NAAT has poor sensitivity for extrapulmonary TB in comparison to pulmonary TB and needs clinical correlation [77]. While LPAs provide rapid detection of drug resistance in TB, their scope is limited to smear-positive samples and identifying specific mutations associated with resistance to key TB drugs such as rifampicin and isoniazid [78]. However, they do not detect all possible resistance mutations, particularly those related to second-line drugs like fluoroquinolones and injectables. This limitation means that while LPAs can confirm resistance to some drugs, they may miss other forms of resistance, necessitating additional testing with more comprehensive methods like culture-based drug susceptibility testing or next-generation sequencing. LPAs done from culture work well for diagnosing extrapulmonary TB or TB in patients with low bacterial loads, such as those co-infected with HIV [79]. MGIT 960 culture, unless repeated with drugs, does not offer a drug resistance profile and requires drug powders, preparation of drugs at specified concentrations, and technical expertise for drug susceptibility testing. For NGS, an elaborate scope is available for comprehensive drug resistance profiling, though data management and bioinformatic analysis are critical.

3.2.6 Trained personnel and human resource constraints

The operation and maintenance of the NAAT machines require specialized skills, but many regions with a high TB burden face a shortage of adequately trained healthcare and laboratory professionals [80]. Limited access to proper training, high staff turnover, and insufficient opportunities for ongoing professional development exacerbate the problem. With Truenat, there is an additional pipetting step, which is particularly problematic in rural or remote areas where healthcare systems often face shortages of skilled workers. In such settings, available healthcare personnel may lack specialized training in molecular diagnostics, leading to improper sample handling or incorrect device operation. The need for continuous training, supervision, and

DOI: http://dx.doi.org/10.5772/intechopen.1007701

support adds pressure on already strained healthcare systems. Interpreting LPA results requires a high level of expertise, presenting a challenge for widespread adoption. The assay results depend on detecting specific genetic mutations, with interpretation involving analyzing hybridization patterns on the test strips. Incorrect interpretation can lead to misdiagnoses, either by falsely identifying drug resistance or failing to detect it when present. Laboratory personnel need specialized training to interpret LPA results accurately, but such training is often unavailable in many resource-limited settings [81]. The handling of mycobacterial cultures poses biosafety concerns due to the infectious nature of MTB and some NTM species. Laboratories must implement strict biosafety measures to protect personnel and prevent the spread of infection. This includes working in Biosafety Level 3 (BSL-3) facilities for MTB cultures requiring specialized equipment and training. Identifying MGIT-positive cultures as MTB and NTM requires correct interpretation and technician expertise. Concerning WGS and tNGS, they need the utmost training and skillset in handling microquantities of DNA and reagents in library preparation and normalization while requiring sound technical knowledge and expertise.

3.2.7 *Quality control and standardization*

Quality control and standardization are significant challenges in deploying the NAATs, particularly in decentralized and resource-limited settings. Ensuring consistent performance across multiple testing sites requires adherence to standardized procedures, which can be difficult to maintain in rural areas with limited supervision. Variability in test procedures, from sample collection to reagent preparation and machine operation, can lead to inconsistent or inaccurate results. This inconsistency is particularly concerning in environments where healthcare workers may lack advanced training in molecular diagnostics. Routine quality control measures, such as external quality assessments (EQA) and internal quality control (IQC), are essential for monitoring test accuracy and reliability [82, 83]. However, establishing these quality assurance programs can be challenging in low-resource settings due to logistical constraints, lack of trained personnel, or inadequate funding. Without robust quality control mechanisms, the reliability of NAAT results can be compromised,

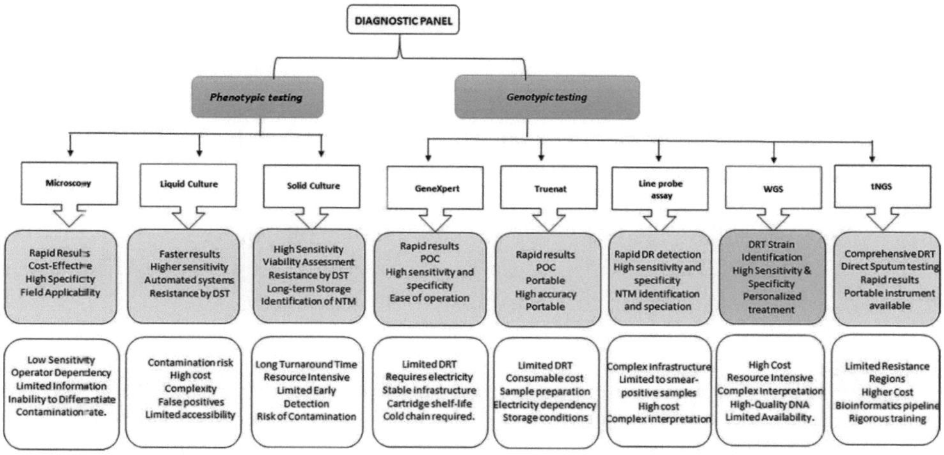

Figure 1.
The advantages and disadvantages of the conventional diagnostic panel.

undermining its effectiveness in TB control. Ensuring proper standardization and regular quality monitoring across testing sites is crucial for maintaining the accuracy and credibility of Truenat-based TB diagnoses. While routine EQAs and IQCs are in place for smear, NAAT, LPA, MGIT, WGS, and tNGS require proper QC checks at various levels. It is done at every lab as per the lab SOP, but no external quality assurance is in place and is a pre-requisite. The various advantages and disadvantages of the available techniques have been shown in the **Figure 1**.

4. Conclusion

Tuberculosis (TB) remains a significant global health challenge, particularly in low- and middle-income countries, despite being one of the oldest diseases known to humanity. While effective treatments exist, the morbidity and mortality associated with TB persist. Recent advancements in molecular diagnostics, particularly nucleic acid amplification tests (NAAT) such as polymerase chain reaction (PCR), have revolutionized TB detection, enabling faster and more accurate diagnosis. This chapter emphasizes the importance of both traditional and modern diagnostic methods, highlighting the complexities and challenges in TB diagnosis. Understanding these advancements is crucial for improving TB management and moving closer to the goal of a TB-free world.

Author details

Radha Gopalaswamy, Gowsalya Saminathan, Vasudevan Manoharan
and Siva Kumar Shanmugam*
Department of Bacteriology, Indian Council of Medical Research (ICMR)-National Institute for Research in Tuberculosis, Chennai, Tamil Nadu, India

*Address all correspondence to: shanmugamsiva27@gmail.com

References

[1] Buzic I, Giuffra V. The paleopathological evidence on the origins of human tuberculosis: A review. Journal of Preventive Medicine and Hygiene. 2020;**61**(1 Suppl 1):E3

[2] Harries AD, Kumar AMV, Satyanarayana S, Takarinda KC, Timire C, Dlodlo RA. Treatment for latent tuberculosis infection in low- and middle-income countries: Progress and challenges with implementation and scale-up. Expert Review of Respiratory Medicine. 2020;**14**(2):195-208. DOI: 10.1080/17476348.2020.1694907

[3] Global Tuberculosis Report 2023. [Online]. Available from: https://www.who.int/teams/global-tuberculosis-programme/tb-reports/global-tuberculosis-report-2023 [Accessed: September 29, 2024]

[4] Lee SH. Tuberculosis infection and latent tuberculosis. Tuberculosis and Respiratory Diseases (Seoul). 2016;**79**(4):201-206. DOI: 10.4046/TRD.2016.79.4.201

[5] Nyirenda T, Moon SY, Jang S, Choe J, Yu SH, Chung D, et al. Call for integration of screening of other respiratory diseases of epidemic potential in TB traditional clinics. Medical Research Archives. 2023;**11**(5)

[6] KS, BTB. Latent tuberculosis infection: An overview. Canada Communicable Disease Report. 2017;**43**(3-4):62-66. DOI: 10.14745/CCDR.V43I34A01

[7] Sharma SK, Upadhyay V. Epidemiology, diagnosis & treatment of non-tuberculous mycobacterial diseases. Indian Journal of Medical Research. 2020;**152**(3):185-226

[8] Gopalaswamy R, Dusthackeer VNA, Kannayan S, Subbian S. Extrapulmonary tuberculosis—An update on the diagnosis, treatment and drug resistance. Journal of Respiration. 2021;**1**:141-164. DOI: 10.3390/jor1020015

[9] Daley CL et al. Treatment of nontuberculous mycobacterial pulmonary disease: An official ATS/ERS/ESCMID/IDSA clinical practice guideline. The European Respiratory Journal. 2020;**56**(1):E1-E36. DOI: 10.1183/13993003.00535-2020

[10] Chopra KK, Sidiq Z, Hanif M, Dwivedi KK. Advances in the diagnosis of tuberculosis-Journey from smear microscopy to whole genome sequencing. Indian Journal of Tuberculosis. 2020;**67**(4):S61-S68

[11] Kassa GM, Merid MW, Muluneh AG, Wolde HF. Comparing the impact of genotypic based diagnostic algorithm on time to treatment initiation and treatment outcomes among drug-resistant tuberculosis patients in Amhara region, Ethiopia. PLoS One. 2021;**16**(2):e0246938

[12] Pagaduan JV, Altawallbeh G. Advances in TB testing. In: Advances in Clinical Chemistry. Vol. 115. Elsevier; 2023. pp. 33-62

[13] García JI, Allué-Guardia A, Tampi RP, Restrepo BI, Torrelles JB. New developments and insights in the improvement of *mycobacterium tuberculosis* vaccines and diagnostics within the end TB strategy. Current Epidemiology Reports. 2021;**8**(2):33-45. DOI: 10.1007/S40471-021-00269-2

[14] Angayarkanni B, Kumar S, Saadhali SA, Azger Dusthackeer VN.

Advancement in the molecular diagnosis of tuberculosis. In: Translational Research in Biomedical Sciences: Recent Progress and Future Prospects. Singapore: Springer Nature Singapore; 2024. pp. 191-205

[15] Mugwagwa T, Abubakar I, White PJ. Using molecular testing and whole-genome sequencing for tuberculosis diagnosis in a low-burden setting: A cost-effectiveness analysis using transmission-dynamic modelling. Thorax. 2021;**76**(3):281-291

[16] Davis JL. Diagnosis of active pulmonary tuberculosis. In: Clinical Tuberculosis. CRC Press; 2020. pp. 115-128

[17] Barletta RG, Steffen DJ. Mycobacteria. Veterinary Microbiology. 2022:345-359

[18] Arora D, Dhanashree B. Utility of smear microscopy and GeneXpert for the detection of Mycobacterium tuberculosis in clinical samples. Germs. 2020;**10**(2):81

[19] Vilchèze C. Mycobacterial cell wall: A source of successful targets for old and new drugs. Applied Sciences. 2020;**10**(7):2278

[20] Khullar M, Oberoi L, Pandhi N. Comparative evaluation of different staining techniques for diagnosis of pulmonary tuberculosis. International Journal of Current Research and Review. 2020;**12**(21):85

[21] Hussey MA, Zayaitz A. Acid-Fast Stain Protocols. American Society for Microbiology; 2008. pp. 1-2

[22] Masali H, Takpere A, Shahapur P. A comparative study of Ziehl-Neelsen stain and fluorescent stain microscopy in the diagnosis of pulmonary tuberculosis. Journal of Pure and Applied Microbiology. 2021;**15**(4):2027. [Online]. Available from: https://digitallibrary.bldedu.ac.in/bitstream/123456789/4119/1/119_2021.pdf [Accessed: September 28, 2024]

[23] Zaporojan N, Anamaria Negrean R, Hodis R, Zaporojan C, Csep A, Carmen Zaha D. Evolution of laboratory diagnosis of tuberculosis. Clinics and Practice. 2024, 2024;**14**:388-416. DOI: 10.3390/clinpract14020030

[24] Wallace E et al. Culturing Mycobacteria. Methods in Molecular Biology. 2021;**2314**:1-58. DOI: 10.1007/978-1-0716-1460-0_1

[25] Pfyffer GE, Wittwer F. Incubation time of mycobacterial cultures: How long is long enough to issue a final negative report to the clinician? Journal of Clinical Microbiology. 2012;**50**(12):4188-4189. DOI: 10.1128/JCM.02283-12

[26] Cook GM, Berney M, Gebhard S, Heinemann M, Cox RA, Danilchanka O, et al. Physiology of mycobacteria. Advances in Microbial Physiology. 2009;**55**:81-319

[27] Procop GW, Roberts GD. Laboratory diagnosis and susceptibility testing. In: Tuberculosis and Nontuberculous Mycobacterial Infections. 2021. pp. 66-74

[28] Rai R, Gautam P, Mathew BJ, Dubey CK, Siddiqui S, Gupta S, et al. Different methods of microscopic and bacteriological diagnosis of tuberculosis. In: Diagnosis of Mycobacterium. Singapore: Springer Nature Singapore; 2023. pp. 51-64

[29] Rupasinghe P, Vereecken J, Graulus P, Decroo T, Ardizzoni E, Hewison C, et al. Middlebrook 7h11 reduces invalid results and turnaround time of phenotypic drug-susceptibility testing of M.

tuberculosis. The International Journal of Mycobacteriology. 2022;**11**(4):407-411

[30] Katila ML, Katila P, Erkinjuntti-Pekkanen R. Accelerated detection and identification of mycobacteria with MGIT 960 and COBAS AMPLICOR systems. Journal of Clinical Microbiology. 2000;**38**(3):960-964. DOI: 10.1128/JCM.38.3.960-964.2000

[31] Su S et al. Diagnostic performance of the metagenomic next-generation sequencing in lung biopsy tissues in patients suspected of having a local pulmonary infection. BMC Pulmonary Medicine. 2022;**22**(1):2020. DOI: 10.1186/s12890-022-01912-4

[32] Böttger EC. The ins and outs of Mycobacterium tuberculosis drug susceptibility testing. Clinical Microbiology and Infection. 2011;**17**(8):1128-1134

[33] Technical manual for drug susceptibility testing of medicines used in the treatment of tuberculosis. [Online]. Available from: https://www.who.int/publications/i/item/9789241514842 [Accessed: September 29, 2024]

[34] Sharma B, Pal N, Malhotra B, Vyas L. Evaluation of a rapid differentiation test for Mycobacterium tuberculosis from other mycobacteria by selective inhibition with p-nitrobenzoic acid using MGIT 960. Journal of Laboratory Physicians. 2010;**2**(02):089-092

[35] Giampaglia CM, Martins MC, Inumaru VT, Butuem IV, Telles MA. Evaluation of a rapid differentiation test for the Mycobacterium tuberculosis complex by selective inhibition with ρ-nitrobenzoic acid and thiophene-2-carboxylic acid hydrazide. The International Journal of Tuberculosis and Lung Disease. 2005;**9**(2):206-209

[36] Bartolomeu-Gonçalves G, Souza JM, Fernandes BT, Spoladori LF, Correia GF, Castro IM, et al. Tuberculosis diagnosis: Current, ongoing, and future approaches. Diseases. 2024;**12**(9):202

[37] Sharma MK, Wonitowy Q, Soualhine H. Conventional and modern approaches for clinical and laboratory diagnosis of tuberculosis. In: Biomedical Translational Research: From Disease Diagnosis to Treatment. Singapore: Springer Nature Singapore; 2022. pp. 209-236

[38] Qin L et al. Dependence of xpert MTB/RIF accuracy for detecting rifampin resistance in bronchoalveolar lavage fluid on bacterial load: A retrospective study in Beijing, China. Infection and Drug Resistance. 2021;**14**:2429-2435. DOI: 10.2147/IDR.S307488

[39] Ngabonziza JC, Decroo T, Migambi P, Habimana YM, Van Deun A, Meehan CJ, et al. Prevalence and drivers of false-positive rifampicin-resistant Xpert MTB/RIF results: A prospective observational study in Rwanda. The Lancet Microbe. 2020;**1**(2):e74-e83

[40] Shea J, Halse TA, Kohlerschmidt D, Lapierre P, Modestil HA, Kearns CH, et al. Low-level rifampin resistance and rpoB mutations in Mycobacterium tuberculosis: An analysis of whole-genome sequencing and drug susceptibility test data in New York. Journal of Clinical Microbiology. 2021;**59**(4):10-128

[41] Nandlal L, Perumal R. Rapid molecular assays for the diagnosis of drug-resistant tuberculosis. Infection and Drug Resistance. 2022;**15**:4971-4984. DOI: 10.2147/IDR.S381643

[42] Sharma K, Sharma M, Modi M, Singla N, Sharma A, Sharma N, et al. Comparative analysis of truenat™ MTB plus and xpert® ultra in diagnosing tuberculous meningitis. The International Journal of Tuberculosis and Lung Disease. 2021;**25**(8):626-631

[43] Jose RA, Inbaraj LR, Vincent RC, Baskar A, Mathew R. Diagnostic accuracy of truenat MTB plus for the detection of pulmonary and extrapulmonary tuberculosis. Indian Journal of Medical Microbiology. 2024;**51**:100709

[44] Dudnyk A et al. Impact of line probe assay-based molecular testing on individualized treatment in patients with rifampicin-resistant tuberculosis: Data from the prospective INNOVA4TB cohort study in Ukraine. Therapeutic Advances in Respiratory Disease. 2024;**18**:1-18. DOI: 10.1177/17534666241249841

[45] Acharya B et al. Advances in diagnosis of tuberculosis: An update into molecular diagnosis of *Mycobacterium tuberculosis*. Molecular Biology Reports. 2020;**47**(5):4065-4075. DOI: 10.1007/S11033-020-05413-7

[46] PMDT – Central Tuberculosis Division. [Online]. Available from: https://tbcindia.mohfw.gov.in/pmdt/ [Accessed: September 29, 2024]

[47] Line probe assays for detection of drug-resistant tuberculosis: Interpretation and reporting manual for laboratory staff and clinicians. 2022

[48] Kim J et al. Comparison of the genedia MTB/NTM detection kit and anyplex plus MTB/NTM detection kit for detection of *Mycobacterium tuberculosis* complex and. Journal of Clinical Laboratory Analysis. 2020;**34**(1):23021. DOI: 10.1002/jcla.23021

[49] Shin S, Yoo IY, Shim HJ, Kang OK, Jhun BW, Koh WJ, et al. Diagnostic performance of the GENEDIA MTB/NTM detection Kit for detecting Mycobacterium tuberculosis and nontuberculous mycobacteria with sputum specimens. Annals of Laboratory Medicine. 2020;**40**(2):169-173

[50] Beviere M, Reissier S, Penven M, Dejoies L, Guerin F, Cattoir V, et al. The role of next-generation sequencing (NGS) in the management of tuberculosis: Practical review for implementation in routine. Pathogens. 2023;**12**(8):978

[51] Colman RE, Mace A, Seifert M, Hetzel J, Mshaiel H, Suresh A, et al. Whole-genome and targeted sequencing of drug-resistant Mycobacterium tuberculosis on the iSeq100 and MiSeq: A performance, ease-of-use, and cost evaluation. PLoS Medicine. 2019;**16**(4):e1002794

[52] Bonnet I, Enouf V, Morel F, Ok V, Jaffré J, Jarlier V, et al. A comprehensive evaluation of GeneLEAD VIII DNA platform combined to Deeplex Myc-TB® assay to detect in 8 days drug resistance to 13 antituberculous drugs and transmission of Mycobacterium tuberculosis complex directly from clinical samples. Frontiers in Cellular and Infection Microbiology. 2021;**11**:707244

[53] Sibandze DB, Kay A, Dreyer V, Sikhondze W, Dlamini Q, DiNardo A, et al. Rapid molecular diagnostics of tuberculosis resistance by targeted stool sequencing. Genome Medicine. 2022;**14**(1):52

[54] Cabibbe AM, Spitaleri A, Battaglia S, Colman RE, Suresh A, Uplekar S, et al. Application of targeted next-generation sequencing assay on a portable sequencing platform for culture-free detection of drug-resistant tuberculosis

from clinical samples. Journal of Clinical Microbiology. 2020;**58**(10):10-128

[55] Barnard M, Parsons L, Miotto P, Cirillo D, Feldmann K, Gutierrez C, et al. Molecular detection of drug-resistant tuberculosis by line probe assay. UNITAID-Expand Project. 2012

[56] Walker FM, Hsieh K. Advances in directly amplifying nucleic acids from complex samples. Biosensors. 2019;**9**(4):117

[57] Ndlangalavu G. Diagnostic accuracy of novel sputum and non-sputum-based tuberculosis diagnostics in HIV-positive patients initiating anti-retroviral therapy

[58] Ardizzoni E. Improved diagnosis of drug-resistant tuberculosis: From implementation of simple phenotypic testing to whole genome sequencing [Doctoral dissertation]. University of Antwerp

[59] Wang L et al. Machine learning analysis of SERS fingerprinting for the rapid determination of *Mycobacterium tuberculosis* infection and drug resistance. Computational and Structural Biotechnology Journal. 2022;**20**:5364-5377

[60] Tang JW, Yuan Q, Wen XR, Usman M, Tay AC, Wang L. Label-free surface-enhanced Raman spectroscopy coupled with machine learning algorithms in pathogenic microbial identification: Current trends, challenges, and perspectives. Interdisciplinary Medicine. 2024:e20230060

[61] Usman M et al. Recent advances in surface enhanced Raman spectroscopy for bacterial pathogen identifications. Journal of Advanced Research. 2023;**51**:91-107

[62] Forbes BA, Hall GS, Miller MB, Novak SM, Rowlinson MC, Salfinger M, et al. Practical guidance for clinical microbiology laboratories: Mycobacteria. Clinical Microbiology Reviews. 2018;**31**(2):10-128

[63] Daum LT, Worthy SA, Yim KC, Nogueras M, Schuman RF, Choi YW, et al. A clinical specimen collection and transport medium for molecular diagnostic and genomic applications. Epidemiology & Infection. 2011;**139**(11):1764-1773

[64] Schito M, Peter TF, Cavanaugh S, Piatek AS, Young GJ, Alexander H, et al. Opportunities and challenges for cost-efficient implementation of new point-of-care diagnostics for HIV and tuberculosis. Journal of Infectious Diseases. 2012;**205**(suppl_2):S169-S180

[65] GLI guide to TB specimen referral systems and integrated networks – stop TB partnership. [Online]. Available from: https://www.stoptb.org/gli-guide-to-tb-specimen-referral-systems-and-integrated-networks [Accessed: September 29, 2024]

[66] Goma R et al. Losses in the sputum specimen referral cascade in Mpulungu District, Zambia: A cross-sectional study. International Journal of Environmental Research and Public Health. 2022;**19**:1621. DOI: 10.3390/ijerph19031621

[67] Marahatta SB et al. Barriers in the access, diagnosis and treatment completion for tuberculosis patients in central and western Nepal: A qualitative study among patients, community. PLoS One. 2020;**15**(1):2020. DOI: 10.1371/journal.pone.0227293

[68] Zhan L, Wang J, Wang L, Qin C. The correlation of drug resistance and virulence in *Mycobacterium tuberculosis*. Biosafety and Health. 2020;**2**(1):18-24

[69] Issadore D, Westervelt RM, editors. Point-of-Care Diagnostics on a Chip. Springer Science & Business Media; 2013

[70] Huggett JF, O'Sullivan DM, Cowen S, Cleveland MH, Davies K, Harris K, et al. Ensuring accuracy in the development and application of nucleic acid amplification tests (NAATs) for infectious disease. Molecular Aspects of Medicine. 2024;**97**:101275

[71] Orikiriza P. Improving diagnosis of childhood tuberculosis in a high TB-HIV prevalent setting [Doctoral dissertation]. Université Montpellier

[72] Xiong XS, Zhang XD, Yan JW, Huang TT, Liu ZZ, Li ZK, et al. Identification of Mycobacterium tuberculosis resistance to common antibiotics: An overview of current methods and techniques. Infection and Drug Resistance. 2024:1491-1506

[73] Nadeem Z, Iqbal J, Kausar S, Noor S, Khan FS, Saleem I, et al. Comparative analysis of the efficacies of the GeneXpert and solid culture media techniques in the diagnosis of mycobacterium tuberculosis. Archives of Razi Institute. 2022;**77**(6):2065

[74] Raizada N, Sachdeva KS, Malhotra B, Thakur R, Kishore Reddy VC. Proficiency assessment mechanism for line-probe assay testing for diagnosis of multidrug-resistant tuberculosis in India. International Journal of Pathology and Clinical Research. 2015;**1**(004)

[75] Cattamanchi A, Miller CR, Tapley A, Haguma P, Ochom E, Ackerman S, et al. Health worker perspectives on barriers to delivery of routine tuberculosis diagnostic evaluation services in Uganda: A qualitative study to guide clinic-based interventions. BMC Health Services Research. 2015;**15**(1):10

[76] Ramasamy P, Sounderrajan V, Harshavardhan S. Current perceptionson advanced molecular diagnostics for drug-resistant Mycobacterium tuberculosis. Biomedical and Pharmacology Journal. 2021;**14**(3):1249-1257

[77] Chopra KK, Singh S. Tuberculosis: Newer diagnostic tests: Applications and limitations. Indian Journal of Tuberculosis. 2020;**67**(4):S86-S90

[78] Yusoof KA, García JI, Schami A, Garcia-Vilanova A, Kelley HV, Wang SH, et al. Tuberculosis phenotypic and genotypic drug susceptibility testing and immunodiagnostics: A review. Frontiers in Immunology. 2022;**13**:870768

[79] Musisi E. Evaluation of the tuberculosis-molecular bacterial load assay for tuberculosis diagnosis and monitoring response to standard anti-tuberculosis therapy [Doctoral dissertation]. University of St Andrews

[80] Engel N et al. Rapid molecular tests for tuberculosis and tuberculosis drug resistance: A qualitative evidence synthesis of recipient and provider views. Cochrane Database of Systematic Reviews. 2022;**4**:2022. DOI: 10.1002/14651858.CD014877.PUB2/ABSTRACT

[81] MacLean EL. Expanding the Use Cases of Molecular Testing for Tuberculosis. Canada: McGill University; 2022

[82] Abebaw Y, Kebede A, Eshetu K, Tesfaye E, Tadesse M, Sinshaw W, et al. Quality assurance practices in tuberculosis diagnostic health facilities in Ethiopia. PLoS One. 2022;**17**(6):e0269601

[83] Shiferaw M. Evaluation of continuous quality improvement of tuberculosis and HIV diagnostic services in Amhara Public Health Institute, Ethiopia. PLoS One. 2020;**15**(3):2020. DOI: 10.1371/journal.pone.0230532

Chapter 7

Treatment Strategies for *Mycobacterium tuberculosis* Infection

Sinazo Cobongela and Tintswalo Mgwenya

Abstract

Tuberculosis (TB), caused by *Mycobacterium tuberculosis* (MTB), remains a critical global health issue, with 1.3 million deaths reported in 2022. Despite available treatments, TB's high morbidity and mortality rates, particularly in low- and middle-income countries, are exacerbated by the emergence of drug-resistant (DR) strains. The limitations of conventional treatments, which rely on older drugs developed over 40 years ago, highlight the need for advanced treatment strategies. Recent advancements include the development and approval of new drugs, such as Bedaquiline (BDQ), Delamanid (DLM), and Pretomanid (PA), which offer novel mechanisms of action against resistant strains. BDQ, a diarylquinoline, inhibits mycobacterial adenosine triphosphate (ATP) synthase, while DLM, a nitroimidazole-oxazole, disrupts mycolic acid synthesis in the bacterial cell wall. Pretomanid targets replicating and non-replicating bacteria by interfering with mycolic acid synthesis and generating reactive nitrogen species (RNS). The introduction of these drugs, particularly in combination regimens such as the six-month Bedaquiline, Pretomanid, and Linezolid (BPaL) regimen, has shown promise in reducing treatment duration and improving efficacy for multi-drug resistant (MDR) and extensively drug-resistant MTB infections.

Keywords: tuberculosis, drug resistance, Bedaquiline, treatment strategies, *Mycobacterium tuberculosis*

1. Introduction

Mycobacterium tuberculosis (MTB) causes tuberculosis (TB), a serious infectious disease. It primarily affects the lungs but can also affect other parts of the body. In 2022, TB caused 1.3 million deaths globally, including 167,000 among people with HIV, making it the second leading infectious killer worldwide, after COVID-19 and above-mentioned HIV/AIDS [1]. Despite all the available treatments and regimens, TB remains a major global health threat. It is characterized by high morbidity and mortality rates, particularly in low- and middle-income countries, and is complicated further by the emergence of drug-resistant (DR) strains [2]. Treatment strategies for TB are crucial for several reasons, given the complex nature of the disease, its

IntechOpen

impact on public health, and the challenges associated with managing it effectively. Preventing transmission is crucial because TB is an airborne infectious disease that spreads through respiratory droplets expelled when an infected individual coughs, sneezes, or talks, allowing the bacteria to be inhaled by others [3]. Effective treatment reduces the number of infectious individuals, thereby cutting the chain of transmission.

The bottleneck of TB treatment, especially multidrug-resistant (MDR-TB) and extensively drug-resistant TB (XDR-TB), by conventional TB treatment, has led to extensive research of new antimycobacterium drugs. The treatment of drug-resistant (DR) TB is challenging due to the prolonged duration of therapy, the potential for drug interactions, toxicity, and the significant financial burden associated with treatment. Therefore, there is a critical need to develop drugs that target novel mechanisms, offer improved efficacy, minimize the risk of drug interactions, have a favorable toxicity profile, and specifically target DR-TB. In the past two decades, there have been significant discoveries in the treatment of DR-TB, including the development of new drugs like Bedaquiline (BDQ), Delamanid (DLM), and Pretomanid (PA), as well as shorter and more effective treatment regimens that improve patient outcomes and reduce the risk of resistance [4–6].

2. Importance of treatment strategies for TB

Treatment strategies for TB are crucial in reducing mortality, preventing drug resistance, limiting transmission, and ensuring treatment adherence. Current treatment with suitable regimen combinations can cure most TB cases, significantly reducing mortality and morbidity rates, especially in high-burden countries. Preventing drug resistance is another key point highlighting these strategies' importance. Inadequate or incomplete treatment can lead to DR-TB, which is much harder and more expensive to treat [7]. Standardized treatment regimens ensure proper use of antibiotics, reducing the emergence of MDR-TB and XDR-TB [8]. TB treatment strategies improve patient outcomes; structured treatment strategies, such as directly observed therapy (DOT), ensure that patients adhere to their medication regimen, leading to better treatment outcomes [9]. Monitoring adherence helps prevent relapses and the development of chronic TB.

Individuals are affected by TB during their most productive years, resulting in significant economic losses due to illness, treatment costs, and lost productivity [10]. Effective treatment minimizes these economic impacts by restoring people's health faster, allowing them to return to work. Vulnerable groups, such as people living with HIV, children, and those with compromised immune systems, are at higher risk of developing active TB [11]. Targeted treatment strategies help protect these populations, reducing the disease's overall burden. TB treatment strategies are crucial for meeting global health goals, including the World Health Organization's (WHO) End TB Strategy, which seeks to significantly reduce TB incidence and deaths by aiming for a 95% reduction in TB mortality and a 90% reduction in overall TB cases worldwide, as well as eliminating catastrophic costs by 2035 [12]. Effective treatment strategies are essential for controlling TB and preventing its spread across borders, thereby ensuring global health security. Ongoing treatment strategies contribute to the body of research, improving understanding of TB and leading to innovations in diagnostics, drugs, and vaccines. Continuous evaluation of these strategies helps them adapt and improve over time.

Effective treatment strategies are crucial to control the disease, prevent its spread, and reduce mortality [13]. Clinical treatment strategies for MTB focus on eradicating the bacteria, preventing drug resistance development, and minimizing transmission. The approaches vary depending on whether the infection is drug-susceptible (DS) or drug-resistant, as well as whether the patient has active or latent TB [14]. Key treatment strategies for TB are discussed below.

3. Standard drug therapy: First-line TB treatment

The combination of first-line anti-TB drugs, which were all developed over 40 years ago, remains a fundamental component of TB treatment [15]. The most common type of TB, DS-TB, solely receives the first-line treatment regimen. Isoniazid (INH), Rifampicin (RIF or rifampin), Pyrazinamide (PZA), and Ethambutol (EMB) are the four main antibiotics that are usually used together to treat DR-TB [16]. Patients with uncomplicated DS-TB are required to take multiple antibiotics. The treatment typically lasts for 6 months, with the first 2 months (the intensive phase) involving the four drugs (INH, RIF, PZA, and EMB), followed by a continuation phase with only INH and RIF for the remaining 4 months [5]. This drug combination is used to achieve therapeutic goals by reducing the risk of bacteria developing resistance to a single agent.

The multi-drug approach is essential because TB bacteria can rapidly develop resistance, especially when using monotherapy [17]. The different drugs target various bacterial mechanisms, making it harder for the bacteria to survive and develop resistance [16, 17]. The combination therapy helps to shorten the duration of TB treatment. Historically, TB treatment could last up to 18–24 months [18]. With the introduction of this combination, the treatment duration for DS-TB has been reduced to 6 months [18, 19]. Individuals with a latent TB infection, in which the bacteria reside in the body without causing active disease, may undergo a more straightforward treatment regimen to prevent its progression to an active state [20]. For example, INH alone or INH with RIF may be used. Although the combination is effective, it requires careful monitoring due to potential side effects [20]. INH can cause liver toxicity and peripheral neuropathy, while RIF can lead to liver dysfunction and drug interactions. PZA may cause hyperuricemia and gout, and EMB can lead to optic neuritis [21]. The widespread use of this drug combination is critical in global efforts to control TB. Its effectiveness is one of the key factors that has enabled TB control programs to achieve significant reductions in TB incidence and mortality worldwide. The emergence of DR-TB strains has underscored the critical importance of proper adherence to the first-line drug regimen, maintaining uninterrupted supply chains, and implementing robust public health strategies for monitoring and managing TB treatment. This includes ensuring timely diagnosis, appropriate patient support to enhance compliance, regular drug susceptibility testing, and integrating advanced diagnostic tools to detect resistance early. Strengthening these areas can prevent the spread of resistant strains and improve overall treatment outcomes, ultimately supporting global efforts to control and eradicate TB [8, 22].

3.1 Mechanism of action of first-line TB treatment

Each of these drugs has a distinct mechanism of action that targets MTB. INH is a prodrug activated by the bacterial enzyme catalase-peroxidase (KatG) to give an active antimycobacterium metabolite, nicotinoyl radical [23]. Once INH is activated, it inhibits the synthesis of mycolic acids, essential mycobacterial cell wall components. Disruption of cell wall synthesis leads to bacterial cell death, particularly affecting actively dividing bacteria. Conversely, RIF's active metabolite (25-desacetyl RIF) binds to the beta subunit of bacterial DNA-dependent RNA polymerase, inhibiting RNA synthesis [24]. This action blocks the transcription of bacterial DNA into RNA, which is crucial for protein synthesis and cell replication. Due to RIF's high potency against MTB, several analogs were developed to enhance its pharmacodynamic properties, improving efficacy, reducing the dosing frequency, and minimizing adverse effects. One successful derivative is Rifapentine (RPT), a cyclopentyl rifampin derivative approved by the U.S. Food and Drug Administration (FDA) in 1998 and has similar effects to RIF. It is primarily utilized in shorter treatment regimens for TB due to its longer half-life and potent bactericidal activity [25]. The bactericidal action induced by RIF and RPT targets actively dividing and dormant TB bacteria, making it highly effective in clearing the infection [5, 24].

In addition to INH targeting the cell wall by inhibiting mycolic acid synthesis, EMB also employs a similar mode of action. EMB inhibits the enzyme arabinosyl transferase, which is involved in synthesizing the arabinogalactan layer of the mycobacterial cell wall [26]. This inhibition disrupts cell wall formation and increases cell wall permeability. EMB is bacteriostatic and works synergistically with other TB drugs to enhance their effectiveness [5, 26]. In contrast to the above-mentioned drugs, PZA uses a different mode of action. The mycobacterial enzyme pyrazinamidase converts the prodrug PZA into its active form, pyrazinoic acid [27]. Pyrazinoic acid stops mycobacterial membrane transport functions and energy production, especially when macrophages are infected, and the environment is acidic [27, 28]. PZA is highly effective against semi-dormant MTB in acidic environments, such as those within TB lesions, aiding in reducing treatment duration [19, 29]. Targeting bacteria in these conditions contributes to the sterilization of infected sites by killing dormant bacterial populations [28].

The combined use of these drugs targets multiple bacterial processes simultaneously, reducing the likelihood of resistance development and increasing treatment efficacy [30]. INH and RIF are particularly potent, while EMB and PZA provide additional mechanisms to ensure a comprehensive attack on the TB bacteria [8, 31]. INH and RIF are the most potent bactericidal drugs, killing actively multiplying bacteria [19]. EMB is mainly included to prevent the development of resistance to other drugs, especially in the early stages of treatment [30].

3.2 Treatment regimen for drug-sensitive TB

The combination of all four drugs is the traditional DS-TB treatment referred to as the HRZE regimen, which is usually administered for 6 months and above, depending on patient response. However, there have been new developments in the past few years with shorter treatment duration compared to the standard six-month regimen. The shorter regimens include second-line TB treatment drugs, such as the fluoroquinolone antibiotic Moxifloxacin (MFX). Like RIF, MFX inhibits bacterial transcription and disrupts DNA replication by interfering with the functions of DNA gyrase and topoisomerase IV [32]. This dual mechanism of action makes Moxifloxacin a strong candidate as a second-line treatment for drug-resistant tuberculosis. This includes the four-month TB regimen, consisting of RPT-MFX with other first-line TB drugs (**Table 1**) [33]. The four-month TB regimen has shortened treatment duration while maintaining high efficacy,

Treatment regimen	Duration
First-line treatment **Intensive phase: HRZE regimen** INH; RIF; PZA; EMB	*6 months* Initial phase: 2 months
Continuation phase: HR regimen IHN; RIF	Continuation phase: 4 months
New and shorter regimen **Intensive phase: With MFX** RPT; MFX; INH; PZA	*4 months* Initial phase: 2 months
Continuation phase RPT; MFX	Continuation phase: 2 months
Intensive phase: Without MFX RPT; EMB; INH; PZA	*4 months* Initial phase: 2 months
Continuation phase RPT; INH	Continuation phase: 2 months

Table 1.
DS-TB treatment regimen and duration.

offering improved patient adherence and outcomes. It was endorsed by WHO and other regulatory bodies in 2021 following results from an international clinical trial tuberculosis trials consortium study 31 (TBTC study 31)/AIDS clinical trial group (A5349) [33]. This study paved the way for alternative treatment regimens for patients with low fluoroquinolone tolerance. It led to the development of a four-month TB regimen incorporating RPT and EMB, along with other standard TB drugs, providing an effective option for those unable to tolerate fluoroquinolone-based therapies (**Table 1**).

4. Treatment of drug-resistant TB

When MTB develops resistance to one or more of the first-line TB drugs, it necessitates a specialized treatment regimen tailored to address the specific resistance patterns. In cases of MDR-TB, where the TB bacteria are resistant to INH and RIF, treatment becomes more complex, requiring second-line drugs that are often less effective, more toxic, and require longer treatment durations of therapy (9–24 months) [8, 22]. XDR-TB, which is resistant not only to INH and RIF but also to fluoroquinolones and at least one injectable second-line drug, poses an even greater challenge, requiring the use of newer drugs like BDQ and Linezolid (LZD), along with a more extensive and prolonged treatment regimen [8, 34].

4.1 Standard drug therapy: Second-line TB treatment

MDR-TB is resistant to at least INH and RIF, the two most potent first-line anti-TB drugs [8, 34]. Fluoroquinolones (e.g., MFX, Levofloxacin [LFX]), injectable agents (e.g., Amikacin [AMK], Kanamycin [KM], and Capreomycin [CM]), and other drugs are among the initial additions to the treatment regimen for MDR-TB [8]. While fluoroquinolones target bacterial transcription and DNA replication, injectable agents focus on bacterial ribosomes to disrupt protein synthesis [35, 36]. Other drugs, such as Clofazimine (CFZ), Ethionamide (ETH), and Prothionamide (PTH), are also important drugs that are included in the treatment regimen for MDR-TB. CFZ targets the MTB DNA, leading to the generation of free radicals, which subsequently cause oxidative stress and disruption of bacterial cell wall synthesis [37]. These mechanisms make it a valuable alternative to both INH and RIF. ETH and PTH have similar mechanisms of action, both inhibiting the synthesis of mycolic acids, the same pathway targeted by INH [38, 39]. **Table 2** lists the treatment options for MDR-TB treatment.

4.2 Treatment regimen for XDR-TB

Treatment options for XDR-TB are limited and often require the use of novel or repurposed drugs, prolonged therapy, and a combination of medications. Therefore, the treatment of XDR-TB involves a combination of second-line TB drugs along with newer, more potent agents that introduce novel mechanisms of action (**Table 3**). Cycloserine (CS) is an older antibiotic with a distinct mechanism of action compared to first-line TB drugs, making it valuable when both first- and second-line treatments fail. CS and its derivative, Terizidone (TRD), primarily inhibit alanine racemase and D-alanine, which are crucial for bacterial cell walls [40, 41]. However, CS is not commonly preferred due to its high toxicity and limited efficacy, while Terizidone (TRD) offers reduced neurotoxicity in comparison [42]. LZD is one of the key drugs used in the treatment of XDR-TB, owing to its potent ability to inhibit protein synthesis and its efficacy against strains resistant to other first- and second-line TB medications [43]. It was approved by the U.S. FDA in 2000 and listed by WHO in 2014 as an essential medicine for MDR-TB and XDR-TB.

Type of TB	Resistance	Treatment regimen	Duration
MDR-TB	IHN RIF	*Second-line treatment* **Intensive phase:** LFX/; MFX; PZA; INHh (high-dose); EMB; CFZ; ETH/; PTH; Injectable agents: AMK/KM/CM	*9–12 months* Initial phase: 4–6 months
		Continuation phase: LFX/ MFX; PZA; EMB; CFZ	Continuation phase: 5–6 months

Table 2.
Second-line TB treatment for MDR-TB.

Type of TB	Resistance	Treatment regimen	Duration
XDR-TB	INH RIF At least one of the fluoroquinolones At least one of the second-line injectables	**Intensive phase:** LFX/ MFX; PZA; BDQ; LZD; CFZ; CS/ TRD; ETH/ PTH	*18–24 months* Initial phase: 6–8 months (or until culture conversion)
		Continuation phase: LFX/MFX; CFZ; LZD; CS/ TRD	Continuation phase: 12–16 months

Table 3.
Second-line TB treatment for XDR-TB.

5. New and emerging TB drugs and treatment regimens

Drug resistance patterns require an individualized treatment approach based on drug susceptibility testing. Newer drugs, such as BDQ, DLM, and PA, offer options for treating XDR-TB by targeting different mechanisms of bacterial resistance and improving treatment efficacy [44].

5.1 Bedaquiline

BDQ belongs to diarylquinolines, a group of anti-TB drugs that target subunit C in the F_0 domain of the mycobacterial ATP synthase [45]. Binding of BDQ to subunit C inhibits the proton pump ability of the ATP synthase, which causes subsequent inhibition of ATP synthesis leading to cell death [46]. BDQ was discovered in the early 2000s [47] as the first drug to get approval from the U.S. FDA for the treatment of MDR-TB. The discovery and approval of BDQ marked a significant era in the drug discovery for TB after 40 years of stagnation in TB drug development [48]. BDQ introduced a novel mechanism of action by enabling a more targeted approach to treatment and potentially reducing the duration of therapy for MDR-TB. Before this, the management of MDR-TB relied on a combination of second-line anti-TB drugs, such as fluoroquinolones (e.g., LFX, MFX), injectables (e.g., AMK, KM), and other antibiotics (e.g., CS, para-aminosalicylic acid). However, these drugs were not specifically designed to treat MDR-TB, resulting in prolonged treatment durations of 18–24 months. In contrast, implementing optimized TB regimens containing BDQ has demonstrated the potential to shorten the treatment duration to as little as 6 months [49]. BDQ is regarded as a last-resort treatment for TB, especially in cases of MDR-TB and XDR-TB where conventional first- and second-line therapies have proven ineffective or unsuitable.

BDQ has been the only diarylquinoline with activity against MTB *for almost two decades*. However, recent preclinical investigations of TBAJ-587 have shown an improved potency and potentially better safety profile than BDQ [50]. Furthermore, due to the emergence of resistance to BDQ, TBAJ-876 is currently under investigation for its efficacy against drug-sensitive TB, MDR-TB, and XDR-TB, including strains that exhibit resistance to BDQ [51]. BDQ has also been derivatized to yield analogs with improved pharmacokinetic and pharmacodynamic properties [52]. However, these analogs have not been clinically evaluated and approved. An increasing number of countries are now utilizing BDQ and DLM, the two newer medications approved by stringent regulatory authorities for the treatment of MDR-TB. By the end of 2017, 68 countries reported using BDQ, while 42 countries had introduced DLM. Resistance to BDQ is linked to mutations in the gene encoding the F_0 domain of mycobacterial ATP synthase [53]. Since its introduction as a treatment option for MDR-TB, thousands of patients worldwide have been treated with BDQ [54]. Unfortunately, there have been observed cases of MTB resistance to BDQ, raising concerns and prompting further research into alternative treatments for resistant TB.

5.2 Delamanid

DLM is a nitroimidazole-oxazole derivative (4-nitroimidazole-oxazole), which is a class of antibiotics that inhibit mycolic acid synthesis in MTB, thereby disrupting the bacterial cell wall and leading to cell death [55]. The bacterial cell wall disruption also enhances drug penetration into the mycobacterium. DLM is a prodrug that is activated through the bioreduction of its nitro group by MTB, a process requiring the reduced cofactor F_{420}, the enzyme F_{420}-dependent glucose-6-phosphate dehydrogenase, and the nitroreductase encoded by the gene Rv3547, to produce its antimycobacterial effects [56, 57]. Similar to BDQ, DLM is used in combination with other anti-TB drugs to enhance efficacy in the treatment of MDR-TB. DLM has been shown to enhance treatment outcomes and reduce mortality in patients with MDR-TB, with a typical treatment duration of 6 months when used in combination with other anti-TB drugs [58]. DLM was approved by the World Health Organization (WHO) and the European Medicines Agency (EMA) in 2014, followed by regulatory approvals in several other countries, including Japan, India, South Korea, and others [59]. To minimize the risk of resistance, DLM is used as part of a combination regimen with other effective TB drugs, reducing the likelihood of resistant strains emerging.

5.3 Pretomanid

PA is a bicyclic nitroimidazole-oxazine with antimycobacterial activity against both replicating and non-replicating MTB by disrupting mycolic acid synthesis and generating reactive nitrogen species, making it effective in treating both active and dormant forms of tuberculosis, including drug-resistant strains [60, 61]. PA is a nitroimidazole antibiotic used in combination therapy to treat drug-resistant forms of TB, including MDR-TB and XDR-TB. Since its approval by the FDA in 2019, protomanid has presented significant advancement in the management of these difficult-to-treat TB strains.

5.4 DR-TB treatment regimen with newer drugs

The inclusion of newer drugs shortens the duration of DR-TB treatment by targeting resistant strains more effectively and enhancing the overall efficacy of the regimen, thereby potentially reducing the length of therapy needed compared to traditional treatment approaches. In 2019, the FDA approved the six-month BPaL TB treatment regimen (**Table 4**), which includes the use of some of the newer TB drugs, BDQ, PA, and LZD, to improve the efficacy and effectiveness of the TB treatment

Type of TB	Resistance	Treatment regimen	Duration
MDR-TB XDR-TB	IHN RIF Fluoroquinolones Injectable agents Other resistance	**Individualized combination therapy:** LFX/MFX; INHh; PZA; CFZ; CS/TRD; ETH/PTH; AMK/KM/CM; BDQ; DLM; LZD Imipenem-cilastatin/Meropenem	Until culture conversion
MDR-TB/ XDR-TB	IHN RIF Other resistance	*Recent & special regimens* **BPaL regimen:** BDQ; PA; LZD **Regimen + newer drugs:** BDQ; DLM Other second-line drugs **Regimen + CLB:** LZD; BDQ; CFZ **Pregnant women treatment:** LZD; BDQ; CS Other regimen with less potential harm to the fetus	6–months (BPaL)

Table 4.
Treatment options for MDR and XDR-TB including newer drugs.

regimen [49, 62]. This regimen has transformed the treatment of RIF-resistant (RR)-TB and other forms of DR-TB by shortening the treatment duration and amount of drugs administered. A recent clinical trial involving the BPaL regimen demonstrated that a reduced dose of LZD maintains its effectiveness while significantly decreasing the toxicity associated with higher doses [63].

6. Treatment regimen for latent TB infection (LTBI)

Latent TB infection (LTBI) treatment is a preventive therapy for individuals who do not show symptoms but are at risk of developing active TB [20, 64]. Preventive treatment reduces the risk of progression to active TB. Common regimens include INH that is taken by patients for 6–9 months, RIF given to the patients for 4 months, or INH and RIF taken once weekly for 3 months (**Table 5**) [20, 64].

7. Other strategies for TB treatment and adjunctive therapy

Close monitoring of patients is essential due to the potential for significant side effects and toxicity from second-line drugs. Despite these advancements, TB remains challenging to treat, requiring individualized therapy based on drug susceptibility testing. The DOT is a World Health Organization (WHO)-supported strategy in which a healthcare provider or trained individual watches the patient take their medication [65]. This method ensures that patients stick to their treatment plan, lowering the risk of incomplete treatment and subsequent drug resistance. DOT is especially critical in communities with high non-adherence rates and in areas with a high prevalence of TB. Malnutrition greatly impairs the immune response and worsens TB outcomes; therefore, the use of adjunctive therapies such as nutritional support and corticosteroids is highly recommended. Nutritional support is vital to improve treatment outcomes, particularly in resource-limited settings [66]. In some cases, corticosteroids may be used as adjunctive therapy in TB meningitis or pericarditis to reduce inflammation and prevent complications [67].

Strategies to treat TB through public health and community-based approaches include contact tracing and screening, health education, and community engagement. Identifying and treating individuals who have been in contact with TB patients is essential to prevent the disease's spread. Educating the public about TB symptoms, the importance of adhering to treatment, and the availability of care is crucial for controlling the disease. Engaging community health workers and utilizing local resources can enhance TB treatment outcomes, particularly in remote or underserved areas [68].

Monitoring and managing adverse effects involve regular assessment and intervention to address side effects. Patients undergoing TB treatment require frequent monitoring to identify and manage adverse effects from the medications, such as

Type of TB	Treatment regimen	Duration
LTBI	INH/ RIF/ INH; RPT	6–9 months 4 months 3 months

Table 5.
Treatment options for LTBI.

hepatotoxicity, nephrotoxicity, or peripheral neuropathy [69]. To manage these side effects and maintain treatment adherence, adjustments to the treatment regimen, symptomatic relief, or drug substitution may be necessary [70]. Treatment approaches for special populations are specifically designed for individuals coinfected with HIV, pregnant women, and children. TB is the leading cause of death among those living with HIV, and co-treatment of TB and HIV is complicated by drug interactions, particularly between RIF and antiretroviral therapy (ART) [71]. An integrated approach, timely initiation of ART, and close monitoring are essential. In pregnant women and children, TB treatment requires special considerations to ensure both the safety and effectiveness of the therapy for the mother and child [72]. For example, in pregnant women, AMK is excluded as a treatment option due to its potential harm to the fetus.

8. Conclusion

Despite significant progress in the development and approval of new anti-TB drugs and treatment regimens, tuberculosis remains a formidable global health issue, particularly due to the rise of drug-resistant strains. The introduction of shorter and more effective treatment regimens, such as the four-month regimen with Rifapentine and Moxifloxacin, represents a promising advancement in managing drug-resistant TB. However, challenges persist, including the emergence of resistance to newer drugs and the complexity of treatment, underscoring the importance of personalized therapy and ongoing research. Effective TB management requires a multifaceted approach, incorporating advanced drug therapies, rigorous adherence to treatment protocols, and supportive measures such as nutritional support and DOT. Addressing these challenges through continued innovation and robust public health strategies is essential to achieving global TB control and ultimately eradicating the disease.

Acknowledgements

The authors would like to extend their gratitude to their affiliations for granting them time to contribute to this book chapter.

Conflict of interest

The authors declare no conflict of interest.

DOI: http://dx.doi.org/10.5772/intechopen.1007538

Author details

Sinazo Cobongela[1,2]* and Tintswalo Mgwenya[3]

1 Health Platform, Advanced Materials Division, Mintek, Randburg, South Africa

2 Department of Science and Innovation (DSI)/Mintek Nanotechnology Innovation Centre (NIC), Advanced Materials Division, Mintek, Randburg, South Africa

3 Diagnostic Unit, Health Platform, Advanced Materials Division, Mintek, Randburg, South Africa

*Address all correspondence to: snazozezethu@gmail.com; sinazoc@mintek.co.za

References

[1] WHO Global Tuberculosis Report, 2023 update. 2023

[2] Bloom BR, Atun R, Cohen T, et al. Tuberculosis. In: Holmes KK, Bertozzi S, Bloom BR, et al., editors. Major Infectious Diseases. Washington (DC): The International Bank for Reconstruction and Development/The World Bank; 2017

[3] Chopra KK, Pandey P, Malik A, et al. Infection control and preventing the transmission of tuberculosis in high-risk centres—Recovery shelter for homeless people. The Indian Journal of Tuberculosis. 2023;**70**:158-161. DOI: 10.1016/j.ijtb.2022.11.002

[4] Singh V, Chibale K. Strategies to combat multi-drug resistance in tuberculosis. Accounts of Chemical Research. 2021;**54**:2361. DOI: 10.1021/acs.accounts.0c00878

[5] Alsayed SSR, Gunosewoyo H. Tuberculosis: Pathogenesis, current treatment regimens and new drug targets. International Journal of Molecular Sciences. 2023;**24**:5202. DOI: 10.3390/ijms24065202

[6] Shetty A, Dick T. Mycobacterial cell wall synthesis inhibitors cause lethal ATP burst. Frontiers in Microbiology. 2018;**9**:1898. DOI: 10.3389/fmicb.2018.01898

[7] Tiberi S, Utjesanovic N, Galvin J, et al. Drug resistant TB—Latest developments in epidemiology, diagnostics and management. International Journal of Infectious Diseases. 2022;**124**(Suppl_1):S20-S25. DOI: 10.1016/j.ijid.2022.03.026

[8] Seung KJ, Keshavjee S, Rich ML. Multidrug-resistant tuberculosis and extensively drug-resistant tuberculosis. Cold Spring Harbor Perspectives in Medicine. 2015;**5**:a017863. DOI: 10.1101/cshperspect.a017863

[9] Sazali MF, Rahim SSSA, Mohammad AH, et al. Improving tuberculosis medication adherence: The potential of integrating digital technology and health belief model. Tuberculosis and Respiratory Diseases. 2023;**86**:82-93. DOI: 10.4046/trd.2022.0148

[10] Meghji J, Gregorius S, Madan J, et al. The long term effect of pulmonary tuberculosis on income and employment in a low income, urban setting. Thorax. 2021;**76**:387-395. DOI: 10.1136/thoraxjnl-2020-215338

[11] Swinkels HM, Justiz Vaillant AA, Nguyen AD, et al. HIV and AIDS. In: StatPearls. Treasure Island (FL): StatPearls Publishing; 2024

[12] Satyanarayana S, Thekkur P, Kumar AMV, et al. An opportunity to END TB: Using the sustainable development goals for action on socio-economic determinants of TB in high burden countries in WHO South-East Asia and the Western Pacific regions. Tropical Medicine and Infectious Disease. 2020;**5**:101. DOI: 10.3390/tropicalmed5020101

[13] Kisling LA, Das JM. Prevention strategies. In: StatPearls. Treasure Island (FL): StatPearls Publishing; 2024

[14] Dartois VA, Rubin EJ. Anti-tuberculosis treatment strategies and drug development: Challenges and priorities. Nature Reviews. Microbiology. 2022;**20**:685-701. DOI: 10.1038/s41579-022-00731-y

[15] Larkins-Ford J, Degefu YN, Van N, et al. Design principles to assemble drug combinations for effective tuberculosis therapy using interpretable pairwise drug response measurements. Cell Reports Medicine. 2022;**3**:100737. DOI: 10.1016/j.xcrm.2022.100737

[16] Padda IS, Muralidhara RK. Antitubercular medications. In: StatPearls. Treasure Island (FL): StatPearls Publishing; 2024

[17] Almeida Da Silva PEA, Palomino JC. Molecular basis and mechanisms of drug resistance in mycobacterium tuberculosis: Classical and new drugs. The Journal of Antimicrobial Chemotherapy. 2011;**66**:1417-1430. DOI: 10.1093/jac/dkr173

[18] Larkins-Ford J, Aldridge BB. Advances in the design of combination therapies for the treatment of tuberculosis. Expert Opinion on Drug Discovery. 2023;**18**:83-97. DOI: 10.1080/17460441.2023.2157811

[19] Dooley KE, Miyahara S, von Groote-Bidlingmaier F, et al. Early bactericidal activity of different isoniazid doses for drug-resistant tuberculosis (INHindsight): A randomized, open-label clinical trial. American Journal of Respiratory and Critical Care Medicine. 2020;**201**:1416-1424. DOI: 10.1164/rccm.201910-1960OC

[20] Price C, Nguyen AD. Latent tuberculosis. In: StatPearls. Treasure Island (FL): StatPearls Publishing; 2024

[21] Badrinath M, Chen P, John S. Isoniazid toxicity. In: StatPearls. Treasure Island (FL): StatPearls Publishing; 2024

[22] Jang JG, Chung JH. Diagnosis and treatment of multidrug-resistant tuberculosis. Yeungnam University Journal of Medicine. 2020;**37**:277-285. DOI: 10.12701/yujm.2020.00626

[23] Suarez J, Ranguelova K, Schelvis JPM, et al. Antibiotic resistance in *mycobacterium tuberculosis*. Journal of Biological Chemistry. 2009;**284**:16146-16155. DOI: 10.1074/jbc.M109.005546

[24] Campbell EA, Korzheva N, Mustaev A, et al. Structural mechanism for rifampicin inhibition of bacterial RNA polymerase. Cell. 2001;**104**:901-912. DOI: 10.1016/S0092-8674(01)00286-0

[25] Rifat D, Prideaux B, Savic RM, et al. Pharmacokinetics of rifapentine and rifampin in a rabbit model of tuberculosis and correlation with clinical trial data. Science Translational Medicine. 2018;**10**:eaai7786. DOI: 10.1126/scitranslmed.aai7786

[26] Meyer FM, Repnik U, Karnaukhova E, et al. Effects of benzothiazinone and ethambutol on the integrity of the corynebacterial cell envelope. Cell Surface. 2023;**10**:100116. DOI: 10.1016/j.tcsw.2023.100116

[27] Njire M, Wang N, Wang B, et al. Pyrazinoic acid inhibits a bifunctional enzyme in mycobacterium tuberculosis. Antimicrobial Agents and Chemotherapy. 2017;**61**:e00070-e00017. DOI: 10.1128/AAC.00070-17

[28] Zhang Y, Scorpio A, Nikaido H, et al. Role of acid pH and deficient efflux of pyrazinoic acid in unique susceptibility of mycobacterium tuberculosis to pyrazinamide. Journal of Bacteriology. 1999;**181**:2044-2049. DOI: 10.1128/JB.181.7.2044-2049.1999

[29] Lamont EA, Dillon NA, Baughn AD. The bewildering antitubercular action of pyrazinamide. Microbiology and Molecular Biology Reviews. 2020;**84**:e00070-e00019. DOI: 10.1128/MMBR.00070-19

[30] Lee N, Patel P, Nguyen H. Ethambutol. In: StatPearls. Treasure Island (FL): StatPearls Publishing; 2024

[31] Rabaan AA, Mutair AA, Albayat H, et al. Tools to alleviate the drug resistance in mycobacterium tuberculosis. Molecules. 2022;**27**:6985. DOI: 10.3390/molecules27206985

[32] Hooper DC, Jacoby GA. Topoisomerase inhibitors: Fluoroquinolone mechanisms of action and resistance. Cold Spring Harbor Perspectives in Medicine. 2016;**6**:a025320. DOI: 10.1101/cshperspect.a025320

[33] Dorman SE, Nahid P, Kurbatova EV, et al. High-dose rifapentine with or without moxifloxacin for shortening treatment of pulmonary tuberculosis: Study protocol for TBTC study 31/ACTG A5349 phase 3 clinical trial. Contemporary Clinical Trials. 2020;**90**:105938. DOI: 10.1016/j.cct.2020.105938

[34] Gandhi NR, Nunn P, Dheda K, et al. Multidrug-resistant and extensively drug-resistant tuberculosis: A threat to global control of tuberculosis. Lancet. 2010;**375**:1830-1843. DOI: 10.1016/S0140-6736(10)60410-2

[35] Rendon A, Tiberi S, Scardigli A, et al. Classification of drugs to treat multidrug-resistant tuberculosis (MDR-TB): Evidence and perspectives. Journal of Thoracic Disease. 2016;**8**. DOI: 10.21037/jtd.2016.10.14

[36] Cegielski JP, Chan P-C, Lan Z, et al. Aminoglycosides and capreomycin in the treatment of multidrug-resistant tuberculosis: Individual patient data meta-analysis of 12 030 patients from 25 countries, 2009-2016. Clinical Infectious Diseases. 2021;**73**:e3929-e3936. DOI: 10.1093/cid/ciaa621

[37] Stadler JAM, Maartens G, Meintjes G, et al. Clofazimine for the treatment of tuberculosis. Frontiers in Pharmacology. 2023;**14**:1-8, 1100488. DOI: 10.3389/fphar.2023.1100488

[38] Favrot L, Ronning DR. Targeting the mycobacterial envelope for tuberculosis drug development. Expert Review of Anti-Infective Therapy. 2012;**10**:1023-1036. DOI: 10.1586/eri.12.91

[39] Wang F, Langley R, Gulten G, et al. Mechanism of thioamide drug action against tuberculosis and leprosy. The Journal of Experimental Medicine. 2007;**204**:73-78. DOI: 10.1084/jem.20062100

[40] de Chiara C, Homšak M, Prosser GA, et al. d-Cycloserine destruction by alanine racemase and the limit of irreversible inhibition. Nature Chemical Biology. 2020;**16**:686-694. DOI: 10.1038/s41589-020-0498-9

[41] van der Walt ML, Shean K, Becker P, et al. Treatment outcomes and adverse drug effects of ethambutol, cycloserine, and terizidone for the treatment of multidrug-resistant tuberculosis in South Africa. Antimicrobial Agents and Chemotherapy. 2020;**65**:e00744-e00720. DOI: 10.1128/AAC.00744-20

[42] Hwang TJ, Wares DF, Jafarov A, et al. Safety of cycloserine and terizidone for the treatment of drug-resistant tuberculosis: A meta-analysis. The International Journal of Tuberculosis and Lung Disease. 2013;**17**:1257-1266. DOI: 10.5588/ijtld.12.0863

[43] Singh B, Cocker D, Ryan H, et al. Linezolid for drug-resistant pulmonary tuberculosis. Cochrane Database of Systematic Reviews. 2019;**2019**:CD012836. DOI: 10.1002/14651858.CD012836.pub2

[44] Espinosa-Pereiro J, Sánchez-Montalvá A, Aznar ML, et al. MDR

tuberculosis treatment. Medicina (Kaunas, Lithuania). 2022;**58**:188. DOI: 10.3390/medicina58020188

[45] Koul A, Dendouga N, Vergauwen K, et al. Diarylquinolines target subunit c of mycobacterial ATP synthase. Nature Chemical Biology. 2007;**3**:323-324. DOI: 10.1038/nchembio884

[46] Lobo MJ, Ray R, Shenoy GG. Gaining deeper insights into the surface binding of bedaquiline analogues with the ATP synthase subunit C of mycobacterium tuberculosis using molecular docking, molecular dynamics simulation and 3D-QSAR techniques. New Journal of Chemistry. 2020;**44**:18831-18852. DOI: 10.1039/D0NJ02062A

[47] Andries K, Verhasselt P, Guillemont J, et al. A diarylquinoline drug active on the ATP synthase of mycobacterium tuberculosis. Science. 2005;**307**:223-227. DOI: 10.1126/science.1106753

[48] Mahajan R. Bedaquiline: First FDA-approved tuberculosis drug in 40 years. International Journal of Applied and Basic Medical Research. 2013;**3**:1-2. DOI: 10.4103/2229-516X.112228

[49] Conradie F, Meintjes G, Hughes J, et al. Clinical access to bedaquiline programme for the treatment of drug-resistant tuberculosis. South African Medical Journal. 2014;**104**:164-166. DOI: 10.7196/samj.7263

[50] Xu J, Converse PJ, Upton AM, et al. Comparative efficacy of the novel diarylquinoline TBAJ-587 and bedaquiline against a resistant Rv0678 mutant in a mouse model of tuberculosis. Antimicrobial Agents and Chemotherapy. 2021;**65**:e02418-e02420. DOI: 10.1128/AAC.02418-20

[51] Almeida D, Converse PJ, Li S-Y, et al. Comparative efficacy of the novel diarylquinoline TBAJ-876 and bedaquiline against a resistant Rv0678 mutant in a mouse model of tuberculosis. Antimicrobial Agents and Chemotherapy. 2021;**65**:e01412-e01421. DOI: 10.1128/AAC.01412-21

[52] Tong AST, Choi PJ, Blaser A, et al. 6-Cyano analogues of bedaquiline as less lipophilic and potentially safer diarylquinolines for tuberculosis. ACS Medicinal Chemistry Letters. 2017;**8**:1019-1024. DOI: 10.1021/acsmedchemlett.7b00196

[53] Andries K, Villellas C, Coeck N, et al. Acquired resistance of mycobacterium tuberculosis to bedaquiline. PLoS One. 2014;**9**:e102135. DOI: 10.1371/journal.pone.0102135

[54] Ghajavand H, Kargarpour Kamakoli M, Khanipour S, et al. High prevalence of bedaquiline resistance in treatment-naive tuberculosis patients and verapamil effectiveness. Antimicrobial Agents and Chemotherapy. 2019;**63**:e02530-e02518. DOI: 10.1128/AAC.02530-18

[55] Field SK. Safety and efficacy of delamanid in the treatment of multidrug-resistant tuberculosis (MDR-TB). Clinical Medicine Insights: Therapeutics. 2013;**5**:CMT.S11675. DOI: 10.4137/CMT.S11675

[56] Szumowski JD, Lynch JB. Profile of delamanid for the treatment of multidrug-resistant tuberculosis. Drug Design, Development and Therapy. 2015;**9**:677. DOI: 10.2147/DDDT.S60923

[57] Hurdle JG, Lee RB, Budha NR, et al. A microbiological assessment of novel nitrofuranylamides as anti-tuberculosis agents. The Journal of Antimicrobial Chemotherapy. 2008;**62**:1037-1045. DOI: 10.1093/jac/dkn307

[58] Skripconoka V, Danilovits M, Pehme L, et al. Delamanid improves outcomes and reduces mortality in multidrug-resistant tuberculosis. European Respiratory Journal. 2013;**41**:1393-1400. DOI: 10.1183/09031936.00125812

[59] Liu Y, Matsumoto M, Ishida H, et al. Delamanid: From discovery to its use for pulmonary multidrug-resistant tuberculosis (MDR-TB). Tuberculosis. 2018;**111**:20-30. DOI: 10.1016/j.tube.2018.04.008

[60] Stover CK, Warrener P, VanDevanter DR, et al. A small-molecule nitroimidazopyran drug candidate for the treatment of tuberculosis. Nature. 2000;**405**:962-966. DOI: 10.1038/35016103

[61] Singh R, Manjunatha U, Boshoff HIM, et al. PA-824 kills nonreplicating mycobacterium tuberculosis by intracellular NO release. Science. 2008;**322**:1392-1395. DOI: 10.1126/science.1164571

[62] Zhu H, Zhou X, Zhuang Z, et al. Advances of new drugs bedaquiline and delamanid in the treatment of multi-drug resistant tuberculosis in children. Frontiers in Cellular and Infection Microbiology. 2023;**13**:1-13. DOI: 10.3389/fcimb.2023.1183597

[63] Haley CA, Schechter MC, Ashkin D, et al. Implementation of Bedaquiline, Pretomanid, and linezolid in the United States: Experience using a novel all-oral treatment regimen for treatment of rifampin-resistant or rifampin-intolerant tuberculosis disease. Clinical Infectious Diseases. 2023;**77**:1053-1062. DOI: 10.1093/cid/ciad312

[64] Huaman MA, Sterling TR. Treatment of latent tuberculosis infection-an update. Clinics in Chest Medicine. 2019;**40**:839-848. DOI: 10.1016/j.ccm.2019.07.008

[65] Karumbi J, Garner P. Directly observed therapy for treating tuberculosis. Cochrane Database of Systematic Reviews. 2015;**2015**: CD003343. DOI: 10.1002/14651858.CD003343.pub4

[66] Grobler L, Nagpal S, Sudarsanam TD, et al. Nutritional supplements for people being treated for active tuberculosis. Cochrane Database of Systematic Reviews. 2016;**2016**:CD006086. DOI: 10.1002/14651858.CD006086.pub4

[67] Schutz C, Davis AG, Sossen B, et al. Corticosteroids as an adjunct to tuberculosis therapy. Expert Review of Respiratory Medicine. 2018;**12**:881-891. DOI: 10.1080/17476348.2018.1515628

[68] Cole B, Nilsen DM, Will L, et al. Essential components of a public health tuberculosis prevention, control, and elimination program: Recommendations of the advisory Council for the Elimination of tuberculosis and the National Tuberculosis Controllers Association. MMWR—Recommendations and Reports. 2020;**69**:1-27. DOI: 10.15585/mmwr.rr6907a1

[69] Prasad R, Singh A, Gupta N. Adverse drug reactions with first-line and second-line drugs in treatment of tuberculosis. Annals of National Academy of Medical Sciences. 2021;**57**:16-35. DOI: 10.1055/s-0040-1722535

[70] Massud A, Syed Sulaiman SA, Ahmad N, et al. Frequency and management of adverse drug reactions among drug-resistant tuberculosis patients: Analysis from a prospective study. Frontiers in Pharmacology. 2022;**13**:883483. DOI: 10.3389/fphar.2022.883483

[71] Navasardyan I, Miwalian R, Petrosyan A, et al. HIV–TB coinfection: Current therapeutic approaches and drug interactions. Viruses. 2024;**16**:321. DOI: 10.3390/v16030321

[72] Hui SYA, Lao TT. Tuberculosis in pregnancy. Best Practice and Research. Clinical Obstetrics and Gynaecology. 2022;**85**:34-44. DOI: 10.1016/j.bpobgyn.2022.07.006